2 - 3 TEARS

SUZIE KLIMT

2 - 3 Tears
Copyright © 2021 by Suzie Klimt

All rights reserved. No part of this publication may be reproduced, distributed, or transmitted in any form or by any means, including photocopying, recording, or other electronic or mechanical methods, without the prior written permission of the author, except in the case of brief quotations embodied in critical reviews and certain other non-commercial uses permitted by copyright law.

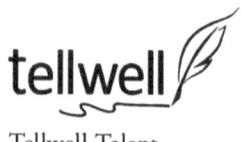

Tellwell Talent
www.tellwell.ca

ISBN
978-0-2288-6099-0 (Hardcover)
978-0-2288-6098-3 (Paperback)
978-0-2288-6100-3 (eBook)

Acknowledgements

I would like to thank my good friend Paula B. for all of the time and effort she put in to help me edit this. Paula, I couldn't have done it without you! You are a true blessing! Thank you for all of your prayers and encouragement!

Thank you also to Janette, Margaret, Jane and Heather for your support and, most of all, your friendship!

Prologue

I am crouched down on the edge of the roof of our two-story home, roughly 25 feet above the ground. The air is thick with the sweltering heat of summer. Beads of sweat run down the insides of my thin little arms as I stare down below me. The sun has kissed the hazy crimson sky goodnight and a warm breeze has picked up, gently caressing my skin, and raising up the hair on my arms. Our neighborhood is quiet but for the gentle humming of cars from the highway in the distance. The sound never sleeps but I have grown accustomed to it and no longer notice it. The shingles are warm and rough against my bare feet as I take rise. Blackbirds perched on a hydro wire nearby are staring at me, their piercing beady eyes, encouraging me. *Jump!* Their shrill metallic-sounding "squee", taunts me. *Jump!* Everything is numb. I feel nothing. All I am aware of is that I must jump. I do not know why. But I am not completely conscious; awake but not aware. I am not even questioning what I am doing here. A strong and heavy magnetic pull brought me here, from the comforts of my bed. There was no choice. No thought was involved. Powerless to resist this force I had climbed up the chain link fence alongside our house and hopped onto the roof, all the while, in a trance-like state. Now here I stood. Toes just slightly over the edge. *Jump! Just do it! You are worthless! No one is ever going to love you. How can they, just look at you! You are ugly*!

Suddenly there is a loud crack of thunder in the distance, and I startle, inhaling sharply. Almost losing my balance, I quickly sit down. Beads of sweat are now trickling down my face. *What am I doing here? Where is everyone? How did I even get here?* I peer down at the ground far below. It has gotten dark, but I can still make out the concrete patio blocks below me. A feeling of terror washes through me. I'm trembling and I don't even think I can stand up. I cannot yell for help because then I will be asked what the heck I am doing up on the roof! How will I answer them if I don't even know myself? No, I will have to keep this a secret. No one must know. Just like the last time this happened, I can't tell anyone. I slide myself back away from the edge and slowly stand up. I can feel my heartbeat racing in my chest. The only way down is to scale the steep sloping part of the roof, then lie on my stomach and search for the top of the fence to rest my feet on. But this is no easy feat because I am only seven years old.

Personality

Oprah Winfrey, Martin Luther King Jr., Carl Jung, and Taylor Swift; we all share the same uncommon personality traits, according to a Myers-Briggs test. Roughly one percent of the population share the traits we share, all of which are walking, talking contradictions! We are easy-going perfectionists. Both logical and emotional, creative and analytical. We often feel misunderstood. For me, that explains things; from a young age, I never felt like I truly fit in anywhere, so I tried to fit myself into a mold of sorts in the hope of feeling more normal.

In general, I do not put too much stock in the whole 'personality type' thing, but reading about it was still somewhat comforting. Though I understand we are all unique in our own special ways, it was reassuring to read that I was not as abnormal as I once believed.

It may sound cliché, but sometimes it feels to me like most of my life was a rollercoaster ride, with no one in the seat beside me to give me a nod of encouragement, or squeeze my hand to let me know everything would be okay.

I have been in counselling multiple times over the years for this. I recently started going to therapy again, but with a new therapist. This woman and I spent the first two sessions going over the highlights of my life, and at the beginning of the third session, she said to me, " You have experienced quite a significant amount of trauma in your life." I looked at her blankly, not knowing how to respond. "How does it make you feel to hear that?" she asked.

Thoughts danced around randomly in my head as I tried to figure out how to respond. When I thought back on my words, it felt like I had told her a tale of someone else's life, and not my own. I wondered, *does this lack of emotion mean that I am detached from my life story? Or have I finally healed from the traumas of the past?*

My mind briefly went fuzzy, until I looked past her outside the window. Beyond the parking lot was a large farmer's field, bordered with a tree-lined fence. I stared at the green of the trees and let my gaze soften. A stillness and tranquility enveloped the land, and it pierced my heart, grounding me.

"I'm at peace with it," I murmured.

In my heart, I know there are so many people who have experienced more significant trauma, and this allows me to just accept my own journey for what it is, and to feel at peace with my past. This peace and inner joy I have within me now came at an extremely high cost with more than a fair share of torment and suffering.

There comes a point in all of our lives when we ask why things happen to us in the way that they do. Often the answer doesn't present itself until long after a particularly difficult life lesson, if at all. It is common to wonder; Why Me? Why was there so much suffering I had to go through? Why did I experience so much torment and pain? Why did the blissful moments seem so brief and end so abruptly, fading to memory among the debris? What did I do wrong? Was it just my fate? Was it part of a bigger destiny? These questions can drive a person mad! Even if we eventually learn the answer, it doesn't change what we must go through. In the midst of chaos, how do we untangle ourselves in order look at the bigger picture? It seems impossible!

I would not change anything that happened to me because I discovered the answers to all those questions. However, before I get there, I have to go back to the very beginning.

Peter

I don't remember much of my childhood. It's like a dark veil blocks it from my consciousness, except for a few pop-up fragments; beyond that, I don't remember most of the first 20 years of my life. Beyond the age of 20, I can recall much more, but even memories of those years feel to me as if I'm watching a movie of somebody else's life. There is a strange detachment in my heart, and a sense that part of it isn't real.

For the most part, to outside observers my childhood looked normal. My younger brother Nick and I played together a lot in our younger years and, like most little brothers, he was a pest. We fought a lot. But I smile when I think about other times with Nick, like the nights we would sing songs in bed, testing the limits of our mother's patience, as we promised her we'd sing 'just one more song' over and over. I would also play cars or Lego with him if he promised to play dolls with me. We would spend hours in the lands of make-believe.

My family lived in a middle-class suburb on a street—Sunnyside Drive—that featured gigantic, lush trees so big they made the roads seem like a tunnel under a canopy of green in the summer months. The 'Sunnyside Gang' consisted of my brother and I, as well as kids of all ages who lived on Sunnyside Drive. In those days, there was no internet and we rarely watched TV;

instead, we spent long, lazy summer days mooching up to people who had swimming pools, making elaborate theater productions, and playing hide and seek until the streetlights came on at night.

The theatre productions were especially fun. We would spend weeks working on plays, making sets and costumes, and then inviting the whole neighborhood to watch our renditions of 'Annie' or 'The Flintstones'. And on those days when we were lucky enough to be allowed into someone's swimming pool, we would lay out our wet towels on the asphalt to sunbathe after a long afternoon swim. I still remember the smell of the hot asphalt driveway.

While every day of summer was an adventure, Fridays were most exciting because that was when we would load up as many empty pop bottles as we could get in a wagon and walk up to the convenience store to redeem them for coins. Ten cents bought a popsicle or a handful of gummy worms. It was much different than it is today; those were times when kids could roam the streets without a care in the world, and it felt safe.

Though we were allowed to roam the neighbourhood with the other kids, Mom and Dad were strict, and not the type to show affection. In fact, I don't remember ever being hugged or hearing, "I love you," from them or anyone until I was an adult. Now it is regularly lavished on me, and I am glad for it. In those days, though, despite our parent's lack of affection, Nick and I were expected to come and greet our father at the door with a kiss on the cheek when he came home from work—no matter what—or we would be in trouble.

When I think back on that now, I wonder, *perhaps they were very loving parents and that part got lost in the fog of my brain.* Who can say, after so many years, what is true and what is the product of an overactive childhood imagination? I do absolutely remember once, when I was in my teens, writing an anniversary card for them. I really wanted to write 'I Love You' on the card, but was terrified to do so because this was not something I had ever said or done before, let alone heard spoken to me.

My family heritage was Austrian. My parents told me that on my dad's side, our family roots traced back to some kind of royalty, so I believed I was part princess—after all, the house my dad grew up in was a huge mansion. Ultimately, it was converted to a red cross mission home of some sort, but I saw pictures of it when it was his family home.

My great-grandfather was a multi-millionaire, and his life makes a most interesting story. During the first World War, the Austrian officer's uniforms were decorated with real gold buttons and tassels. After the war, nobody wanted any reminder of the tragedy and horror of this war, so all the uniforms were heaped on trains to be sent away. The loading of these trains happened to take place in the town where my great-grandfather lived. A shrewd businessman, he saw an opportunity and so he bought the entire trainload of old, bloody uniforms for a dirt-cheap price, removed the gold, melted it down, and was suddenly rich! He used the remaining high quality woven fabric to make gloves, and then sold them to steel manufacturing plants.

Our family owned many homes and buildings throughout Austria, and my great-grandfather—because of his significant financial contributions to the defense effort—once even had an audience with Kaiser Franz Josef. However, when the Second World War came, everything was bombed and destroyed.

My father and his brother immigrated to Canada at the ages of 21 and 28 respectively, following the death of their mother. They came each with only a suitcase in hand, with enough money for three months' rent. My paternal grandfather, who had been a high-ranking officer in World War I, passed away from Malaria when my dad was only one year old. My grandmother suffered not only the loss of her husband, but subsequently the loss of three of her children due to polio. Left with my father and my Uncle Karl, she raised them on her own through famine, bombings, and air raids. I cannot fathom what it must have been like to be wealthy and then suddenly not have food to feed your children.

Growing up during Nazi occupation, Dad was recruited to be an Olympic runner when he was only 14 years old. However, his mother would not let him join because she did not want any association with the Nazis. Dad was also trained to be a concert pianist, but all that ended when he came to Canada and severed the tendon in his hand while working on a farm. Ultimately, he went on to become a senior manager for a large corporation after years of hard work.

Prior to immigrating to Canada, my Dad's brother spent seven years as a front-line soldier. He sustained a bullet wound to the and miraculously he survived. Today he is 97, a world-renowned artist, and fit as a fiddle.

Like my father, my mother's side of the family is of Austrian heritage as well. Her parents were farmers. My grandmother came to Canada on her own when she was just 12 years old. At the time, she didn't speak any English. I cannot even fathom the idea of my children riding the transit system alone at age 12, let alone travelling across continents and supporting themselves in a strange country, all alone. However, as hard to imagine as it is, somehow she managed to get a job, learn the English language, and support herself.

My grandfather on my mother's side was born in Canada, but he was kicked out of his home at the age of ten, leaving school with only a grade two education. Despite this rocky start, he always managed to find work. He was extremely intelligent and was the first Canadian to invent his own solar powered home system. Meanwhile, his own mother decided to pursue her Bachelor of Arts Degree at the age of 82, taking the bus to the university every day.

My mother moved away from the family farm and into the city at eighteen years old. With nothing more than a high school education, she became a radio programmer and later on became a manager at an insurance company.

Ultimately, my bloodline consists of a long line of folks with strong constitutions, determination, imagination, and endurance. These men and women were tough fighters and people who persevered through every imaginable adversity. This is part of my DNA.

As I mentioned, many of my childhood memories are inaccessible to me. However, now and then I remember such childhood activities as setting up blankets beneath the shade of the apple trees in our backyard and playing with my Barbies. Long past the age when most girls had stopped playing with such toys, I would get lost in a world of make-believe. The handsome Ken doll always thought my Barbie was the prettiest of all, and there was always a 'happily ever after'. I held on to that fantasy world until I replaced it with another one—the romance novel. I didn't merely read those novels; I completely immersed myself in them. I was the beautiful woman, and the tall dark handsome man would always fight for my love and go to the ends of the Earth to be with me, and we would live happily ever after. I became convinced that this was my destiny!

But, as I have mentioned, these happy times were the exception and not the rule. My parents did the best they could; they really did. I can say this now after much therapy. They were flawed people, as we all are. My mother came from an abusive home and was raped by a distant, visiting uncle at a young age. My father grew up during the Nazi regime in Austria which made him rigid and somewhat overbearing. Like all of us, they were products of their upbringing, and perhaps this is what rendered them incapable of expressing much emotion, other than anger. Obedience, order, and discipline replaced vulnerability, openness, and compassion in their parenting, and it was Nick and I who paid the price.

As a child, I remember always thinking that their rules were way too harsh. Spilling a drink at the table or laughing with my brother would result in missed meals, a lot of yelling, and criticism. Punishments included everything from being kicked, shaken or struck, to having objects thrown at us, being forced to memorize quotes from the Bible, or having to sing German folk songs. I was called names including 'heathen', 'stupid', and 'devil's child', to name a few. At the time, I did not know what a heathen was, but it didn't sound good.

I was afraid of God. To me, God was this big scary man in the clouds who would punish me in the fiery pits of hell if I misbehaved. I was afraid of my father. When he yelled, the walls shook. When he was angry, he would say that he 'saw red', and I thought that meant my blood, and so I did my best to be an obedient, outwardly happy child. But as well as being deeply frightened, I was deeply angry. Sometimes, in my rebellion, while they were out of sight I would sneak into my parent's bedroom and spit on their beds. It was super scary to go and do that, and I would always feel guilty afterward, but it was the only way I could express the anger that was growing inside and all around me—though it seems pretty crazy now as I write this.

In those days, in our neighborhood, mothers stayed home and cared for the children, house, and garden while fathers worked. Often, the mothers had afternoon tea with each other while we kids played, and there were plenty of trips and outings. Nick and I, like the rest of the neighbourhood kids, had nice clothes, good food, and warm beds. We wanted for nothing—except love. I desperately wanted to feel loved, but instead, I lived in utter fear of doing something wrong to upset someone. I could not express my feelings because my dad, having grown up in an era of 'children are meant to be seen, not heard', would not tolerate seeing his children cry. If he caught us crying, he would tell us we were weak and so, when I was sad, I put a smile on my face and pretended everything was okay. Mom had a temper too, and liked using the wooden spoon, but she did not intimidate me as much as my Dad. What did scare me was the thought of her reporting my misbehavior to him and then having to deal with his wrath. To me, it was beyond comprehension that people could be so mean and angry.

When my father was raging, I would pack a bag and have it ready under my bed in the hope that I would be brave enough to run away. But the next morning I would wake up with immeasurable guilt and fear of my bag being discovered, and so I would quickly unpack it. I also learned how to take apart my window in silence and climb out in less than 30 seconds, but despite my elaborate plans to live in the ravine nearby—and eventually find someone to take me far away—I never made it out of my backyard. Most times I never even made it out the window.

My family occasionally travelled. My favorite vacations were the ones we took to Austria when I was young. Somehow, being away from our family home made me feel better and happier. In Austria, we stayed stay with my cousins in a small village nestled in the mountains. The contrast of the beautiful, lush, flowing, vibrant greenery against the backdrop of the sharp, jagged mountains, still calls to me to this day. If I could have stayed in that village in Austria, I would have. It felt like home to me. My cousins adored me, and my predominant memory is a feeling of contentment and peace. Because of some family business my parents needed to take care of, Mom and I ended up staying there for a prolonged time. I went to part of grade one there, and I remember sitting in class, not knowing how to speak German, but not feeling at all shy. At home, I always felt shy. I didn't want to go home; when we returned, the heaviness that loomed over me returned as well, as did my father and all his anger.

My early years, dominated by fear as they were, left me with a deep yearning to feel loved and noticed. I wanted people to like me, and so I became a people pleaser—the girl who is always happy, full of energy and eager to accommodate. For example, if my friend Kara wanted to sing songs and I didn't, I would sing songs anyway to please her. If my friend Joan wanted to practice makeup and I didn't, I would practice putting on makeup to please her. I did not know how to stand up for myself.

Since I was slightly older than most of the other girls, I thought that acting tougher and wiser would prompt them to like me more, but the harder I tried, the more alone and empty I felt inside. I held a subconscious belief that I had to prove myself to everyone in order to be noticed, which made me highly competitive. I played street hockey with the boys to show how strong I was to all the girls. Any time I ran with other kids, I had to be the fastest. If my friends and I played dress-up in our parents' old clothes, I had to have the best and prettiest outfit. But at that age, I didn't understand that such efforts weren't appreciated by other kids, and so when I did not receive the attention I craved, I would bury the feelings of sadness and unworthiness deep down in my heart where no one could see them.

As a child, I preferred having close relationships with one or two friends rather than being in a group. I loved the feeling of sisterhood I got from sharing darkest secrets and biggest dreams with my friends. In kindergarten, my first 'best friend forever' (BFF) was Emma. Unfortunately, a year later after we met, she moved to New Zealand—and I was crushed. Little did I know this was the beginning of a trend … people leaving. After Emma, I became friends with Amy who, the following year, also moved far away, leaving me to find a new friend.

Then there came Peter. Peter was a sweet boy who lived down the street. He had white-blond hair and sported the ever-fashionable 'bowl cut' hairstyle that was popular at the time. I still remember his freckled, smiling face and he was so nice to me where others showed indifference. I have to hold back tears even now as I write. He was just a genuinely sweet soul and that type of person that people were drawn to.

We were only in grade four so I didn't know what having a crush was, but I suppose you could call it that. With living only a few houses apart, spending all our free time together was easy. He made me smile and I felt so happy just to be near him. With Peter, I felt like I could just be myself, like I didn't have to try so hard to fit in. He just accepted me, quirks and all, without judgement. When grade five came, Peter left the school we attended to start at a French immersion school. It made me sad because I did not really have many other friends at school that I connected with. I really missed him, but every day we would see each other coming home from school. One day, he was not there. I found out later that Peter had been hit and killed by a car less than half a block away.

After my mother told me, I remember locking myself in the bathroom, sitting on the floor with my face buried in a towel so that no one would hear me cry. I couldn't let anyone see my sadness because I had been brought up not to let weakness show. I had to be strong, so of course as soon as I was able, I quickly went back to pretending there was nothing wrong. I also could not bring myself to go to the funeral and see him lying there dead, because death, and the idea of a terrifying God—not to mention the pits of hell—scared me. Unfortunately, not saying goodbye to Peter would ultimately haunt me for years to come. Every time I thought of Peter, I felt guilty; like I should have been there for him in that final way. The dark voices whispered in my ear telling me that I was a coward for not going.

About ten years after Peter's death, I went to visit a psychic. The first thing she told me as I sat down was that there was a young, blond boy with me. She described him as around eleven years old, with white-blond hair and a face full of freckles. I felt the hairs on the back of my neck stand up and got shivers down my spine. Peter! She went on to tell me that he had a message for me. She said, "He told me to tell you that it's okay."

I must have turned white as I related to her how guilty I had felt for not going to the funeral. She said, "He wants you to let go, and he understands. He is not upset. He loves you." After leaving her office, I was not sure what to make of the whole thing;

however, I was finally able to let Peter go, and the guilt I had been feeling was released.

Having a new friend helped me forget the pain of losing Peter. Sanna felt like my sister right from the start. She moved in across the street a couple months after Peter's death, and she was so pretty, with her platinum blond hair and blue eyes. Everyone liked her and wanted to be her friend, but she and I were like two peas in a pod. We did everything together, from dance lessons to sleepovers. When she moved back to Finland a couple of years later, I was heartbroken. I could not reconcile why the few friends that I had, kept leaving me and I felt alone.

Then Joan moved into the neighborhood, and once again I had another best friend. However, we drifted apart halfway through grade eight, when she started to hang around the popular kids. I could not follow her into that group because, even though I tried hard to fit in, I was reserved and quiet, so people tended to ignore me. Even worse was that all the girls in the class seemed to have developed breasts and gotten their periods, and all of them were being noticed by boys except me. Worried that there was something wrong with me, and wanting so badly to fit in, I took to stuffing my bra with cotton balls and lying about having my period.

We all have to face bullies in our lives, in some shape or another. Some of us become the victim; others become the bully; still others become spectators. I, unfortunately, was the one being bullied. As if being the tallest, skinniest person in my class wasn't enough, my nose seemed to grow faster than the rest of my face, convincing me—and others, that I was 'the ugly duckling'.

Now, when I look back at pictures, I can see that I was nowhere near as ugly as I thought. With my long, permed, golden-brown hair and my aquamarine eyes, some may have called me pretty. However, I was so insecure in every aspect of my being that when one boy started calling me 'big nose', I could not bear the shame of it. The name caught on and made its way all through the school, until even some my so-called friends would say it.

All through grade seven and eight I had a secret crush on a boy named Nate. To me, he was the best-looking boy in school, and I knew that there was no way he would ever even look my way. Yet that did not stop my pre-pubescent heart from pining for him. One day Nate was standing with a group of boys who liked to tease me. I dreaded having to walk past them, but there was no way around it. I knew what was going to happen and that they were going to humiliate me again by calling me that awful name. But it was too late, they already saw me coming. My heart was beating wildly in my chest while I held my breath and clenched my sweaty palms. *Please, oh please don't call me that name in front of Nate!* I tried to walk as fast as my long, gangly legs could go, while pretending to be captivated by some scenery in the distance. I almost made it past them, and was ready to let the air out of my lungs, when I heard it: "Hey BIG NOSE, where are you running off to?"

I turned around and smiled at them—and then saw Nate, my crush, laughing with the rest of them. I turned and ran away. As I had been taught to do, I pretended it didn't bother me, but that night, as it happened most nights, my pillow was soaked with tears. I started to wear a swimmer's nose plug to bed at night in hopes that it would shrink the monstrosity on my face but, unsurprisingly, it didn't help.

None knew what was going on inside of me. The world saw a quiet, shy, but happy and kind girl but I had begun to realize that with being ugly, I was unlikely to get the handsome prince and my happy ending that I fantasized about. I still held fast to that dream because somewhere inside me I knew that if I found the love I so desperately craved, everything would be alright.

My daily fight as a child was to shut off the constant voice in my head that told me I was not good enough, smart enough, or pretty enough. Sometimes that voice would utterly consume me for a few hours and I would occasionally fantasize about lying in the middle of the road, just waiting for a car to run over me, because I did not know any other way to shut that voice out. I also had no idea where these dark thoughts and feelings came from, or when they would come; however, once they were spent, they would leave as abruptly as they came. It was all very confusing for me, and I felt lost, terrified, and alone; like no one understood me. There was no way I could share these thoughts and feelings with anyone because I did not want to appear any more different than I already felt. Besides, I was too scared of getting in trouble.

There were happy times, times when I would forget the darkness, like when I was playing with my brother Nick or with my neighbourhood friends, or the times mom would take us on outings. But then, out of nowhere, this urge to end my life would surface like an overpowering tidal wave, and I would find myself perched on our rooftop wanting to jump off. Somewhere inside me, I knew this was not normal but how could I face it at such a young age? It paralyzed me with fear. I didn't want to be different! I knew there was a dark shadow that followed me for as long as I could remember, but there was no way I could tell anyone, so I tried hard to pretend it was not there by distracting myself. Most of the time I was able to pull it off on the exterior. But it was so difficult to pretend that I was just like all the other girls, with this terrible awful black lead weight that inhabited the inside of my body.

At home, in the presence of my parents, I had a hard time understanding why they were always so mean and angry. While we were not allowed to watch much TV (my dad said it was the devil's instrument), the times when we did, I would lose myself deeply in the characters, just as I did when I read my novels. My heart ached to be one of the pretty women who gets her man—and that soon became the goal of my life. I decided that once I was old enough, I would put all I was into finding a man to love me.

Something deep down inside seemed to whisper me that finding this love, would make all the darkness go away.

Of course, I didn't know what love was, but that didn't matter—all I wanted was to feel special to someone, to feel like I mattered to just one person. In elementary school, none of the boys I liked reciprocated my feelings except, perhaps, Peter. I missed Peter. He was my friend. I could only hope that high school would be so much different and better!

Tomas

I held tight to the idea that high school would be better than elementary school for me, but boy was I in for a shock! Once I got there, again I felt invisible and utterly alone. The mean guys who had made fun of me were gone, but somehow I still felt like the ugly duckling. If I could have worn a sign that summed up my high school years, it would have said: "PLEASE will someone be my friend?" in big red letters.

I would not let people look at my side profile, because I didn't want them to notice my nose and make fun of me. I wore a lot of makeup to bring attention to my eyes, so people would be less likely to notice my nose. The dark shadow following me was ever present but I was learning how to distract myself and push it away by being busy. Often, during lunch, I would eat my sandwich in a bathroom stall, or I would go for long walks alone.

I had some people—acquaintances, really—in my life, but I wouldn't say they were real friends. Mostly, I tried to hang around with certain groups and pretend to be like them, but I felt like a fish out of water. These groups accepted me as one would accept a fly in the room, and that felt hollow. I wanted a *true* friend, but people seemed so superficial. In an effort to fit in, I tried to be 'that girl', talking about makeup and hair and clothes, or hanging out at the mall, but it all seemed so insincere. To make matters worse, the battle inside me grew stronger and looking back now, it felt like my soul was constantly being pulled between darkness and light, only I was not aware of this. I only knew that I was different from everyone else. And not different in a good way.

Luckily, Joan and I were still in touch, and we would get together sometimes, so that took the edge off what was going on at high school. One day she invited me to her house to meet her cousins, who had just moved to Canada from Germany. They did not speak English, and she knew I could speak some German, so she wanted me to translate.

I was so excited to meet her cousins. Tomas and Mike were cute and sophisticated, with long, shaggy brown hair, dazzling brown eyes, and European cigarettes. I liked the older one, Mike, because he had this air of confidence about him and looked like he could be on the cover of a Harlequin Romance Novel. I quickly learned that the feeling was not mutual, and so I set eyes upon Tomas. I had not really noticed him before because he was more reserved and quieter. But the more I looked at him, the more I liked him. Something about him reminded me of Peter with his boyish face and spray of freckles across his face. He was very tall and lean and had these huge dimples on his cheeks that I just wanted to kiss! It did not take long for me to fall head over heels in love with him.

Because they were new to the country, they had not yet made any friends and so I was only too happy to accommodate them and be the friend I thought they wanted. As usual, I wanted to fit in with them and so I had to make myself sophisticated too. I got new clothes and started laying on the makeup even heavier than usual, hoping they'd find me acceptable.

I am no longer in touch with Tomas and Mike, but if I was I'm sure they would make fun of me for this story—a story about a girl (me) who has never smoked before.

Mike and Tomas smoked, so of course I had to smoke too. How else was I going to catch their attention? The only problem was that I had never smoked before, so Joan and I went and bought a pack of cigarettes at the corner store so we could practice. During lunch period, we went into the back forest of our school to try. We didn't even know how to light a cigarette, let alone smoke one. We did not know that you have to draw on it at the same time you put a match to it to make the thing ignite, and so we fumbled around until by pure luck we managed to get one going. Then we tried to inhale. Understandably, we ended up coughing and sputtering—however, we were determined to learn to smoke so we kept practicing. Eventually we got the hang of it, and began to think we were pretty sophisticated with our cigarettes.

That night, we were out for a walk in the park when the boys pulled out their smokes. It was our big moment: Joan and I, in our new high-waisted blue jeans, teased bangs and freshly painted nails, pulled out our pack too. The guys watched in amusement as we nonchalantly tried lighting our smokes by holding them in our hands instead of our mouths and attacking the end with match after lit match. Of course, the cigarettes would not stay lit. Finally, Tomas offered assistance, telling us that we had to put them up to our mouths to light them. Mortified and still trying to pretend we were expert smokers, I politely informed him that this was the way we lit cigarettes in Canada! He teased me about this for years.

A few months later, Mike and Tomas moved 50 kilometers away. I was crushed because by this time, I was convinced that Tomas was my prince and my happily ever after—but that he just did not know it yet! However, we kept in touch and regularly talked on the phone. Eventually, I became his confidante and found myself giving him dating advice. He would come to me with his relationship problems, and I would do my best to coach him ... but all the while, my delicate little teenage heart was pining for him.

I don't remember how it came to be, but one day we both skipped school, and went to my house while my parents were at work. I really believed that sleeping with him was the only way to get him to like me the way that I liked him, and so I lost my virginity to him. It was nothing like my romance novels. It was so empty and fast, and afterwards I felt used and alone. To make matters worse, Tomas didn't talk to me for a couple months after that, though eventually we resumed our friendship, and I went back to being his friend and romance coach as if nothing had ever happened.

We would talk on the phone for hours. I was convinced that he would eventually realize that he loved me, but that never happened. Instead, he got into a long-term relationship with a girl who didn't want him talking to me. After that, we had sporadic contact for a few years but we eventually lost touch. I was sad about this because not only had I lost a friend, but it was also goodbye to 'prince number one'.

After Tomas, I felt bereft and unlovable and so when any guy showed the slightest bit of interest in me, I lit up—even when the attention was from someone I had no interest in at all. I was desperate for attention because I could hear this voice inside me telling me how unworthy I was, and that I would never be able to have anyone for my own. But I was still happy Suzie on the outside, going along with what everyone wanted to do, being the doormat, the servant, the pleaser.

I was fortunate that the dancing and competitive swimming I'd practiced throughout my childhood had at least given me a decent figure and so, to draw attention, I highlighted that by wearing sexy clothes. However, my chest wasn't quite as developed as I wanted it to be, and so to compensate I stuffed cotton balls inside my bra to look bustier. Then, all dolled up, I would follow my friends to parties, where I would drink way too much alcohol, even though I never really enjoyed drinking. I thought getting drunk with everyone else was the only way to have friends, and soon it got to the point where every weekend I would be drunk at a party. But still, no one ever noticed me. All I wanted to do was sit and talk with someone, but everyone was interested only in getting high, making out, or playing drinking games. Once in a while it was fun to have the alcohol provide a temporary amnesia from my life, but mostly at those parties, I watched while my friends hooked up with guys, while I ended up alone again. Often I would end up going for a walk or leaving early, with my dark shadow close by.

One day when I was in grade eleven, I was in my religion class when suddenly I was filled with so much sadness that I knew that I had to end my life. A dark, intense feeling, like a detached coldness, washed over me, convincing me that my life was hopeless and that I would never find love. I felt nothing except a desire to end my life. There was no thoughts or emotions in me. It felt I was just a puppet being moved along by some invisible dark force. I went home, tied a belt around my neck, attached it to the upstairs railing, and kicked the chair out from under me. Just like that. It was like I was on autopilot. I felt nothing. I didn't even write a goodbye note. I was in a tunnel with only one exit. Then the belt broke and I came crashing to the ground. I sat there bewildered and dry-eyed for a few minutes, and then cleaned up. I never told anyone, and no one ever found out.

When the family came home, it was business as usual, and no one suspected a thing. It was as if nothing had happened. The feeling I'd had that I had to end my life left me just as quickly as it had arrived. I even pretended to myself that it hadn't happened and I put the whole experience in a box deep inside my mind. It would be almost ten years later, during therapy, before I remembered and acknowledged it again.

Shane

By the time grade 12 came around, I had become more focused on the future. I had spent the previous four years lifeguarding part-time and I had decided that I wanted to be a paramedic. The job appealed to me because it required only two years of schooling. It was even more appealing to me because I was so anxious to move away and start my own life. I firmly believed that once I left home, everything would be better.

I was still quite unhappy. A school, I still ate my lunch alone during my long walks, and I still tried hard to avoid people from seeing my side profile so they wouldn't see my big nose. But the idea of being a paramedic caused me to see a brighter future in doing something meaningful with my life.

As part of a school program, I did a co-op placement in a hospital, in which I excelled. Anatomy and physiology of the human body fascinated me and I really wanted to watch an autopsy. This was definitely not something that was common but after pleading many times, the staff agreed to let me. I did not tell any of my friends, because I did not want anyone to judge me for being so interested in this. Watching autopsies for fun at seventeen is not exactly the 'norm'. I spent a lot of my free time after I had finished my co-op shift, down in the morgue watching the autopsies and asking all kinds of questions about what they were doing. The I had the idea to ask if I could watch a life surgery. There was quite a bit of red tape to go through but finally they said yes!

I was, however, only allowed to observe an arthroscopic knee surgery. At this time in my life, I was having problems with one of my own knees and my family doctor had said he was considering making a referral for me to have the same surgery. I thought it would be exciting to watch a surgery that may be performed on me ... but as soon as they started, I began imagining it was *my* knee being jostled around and I fainted right there in the operating room, in front of all the nurses and doctors, out like a light.

Afterward, I insisted I was okay, and they gave me a chair so that I could watch the rest of the surgery. I was so humiliated that I did not complain about the bump on the back of my head, or the dizziness I was feeling. Needless to say, they never invited me back to watch another surgery and I was too scared to ask; however, this did not deter me from my desire to pursue a career in medicine. Instead of being a paramedic, I dreamed of being a doctor in an emergency room—but I simply could not fathom living at home and spending another eight to ten years in school.

Internally, a tug-of-war was taking place between two very distinct sides of my personality. On one hand, I liked helping people and I wanted to make a difference in the world. That side of me was easy going, adventurous, driven and fiercely loyal to friends, who came to me for advice because I was understanding and empathetic. On the other hand, I kept hidden a part of myself that was shy, needy, and insecure, and who believed that the only way to find true happiness was to find a man to share her life with. For that part of me, happiness and self-worth were completely dependent on the love of a good man, and the fantasy of that perfect, loving relationship. Looking back, it is the longing of *that* girl that would shape the course of my life.

I was barely 17 when I met Shane at a house party. Shane was the football star and the best-looking guy in school. He had these mesmerizing piercing blue eyes and blond hair that would put Vanilla Ice to shame. Shane was the type of guy that everyone gravitated towards because he had this alluring quality to him that demanded attention. At that time, I was working as a lifeguard and when he noticed my lifeguard shirt he used it to spark up a conversation. I told Shane that I wanted to be a paramedic, and explained that I was attracted to the job because it would allow me to work in healthcare, but be done with school quickly.

When Shane heard that I was going to be a paramedic he became very interested in talking more, but I was so insecure that I was stunned he was even talking to me. I couldn't believe it, and I assumed he was just trying to learn more about becoming a paramedic ... and yet I had a crazy notion that he was flirting with me. How could it be?

I loved the attention, and we ended up dancing and talking all night. Later, he asked for my number. He seemed genuinely interested in me and I began to see my happily ever after. He thought Barbara Streisand was one of the most beautiful women in the world, and claimed that I looked like her. Everyone, especially me, was stunned when we began dating.

Things with Shane were magical, but a few months after we started dating, I had to have my tonsils removed. At that time, you were kept overnight in the hospital and when Shane came to see me after surgery, I wasn't wearing any makeup. I inwardly cringed. Up until then, I had never let him even catch a *glimpse* of me without makeup on, and I still tried to avoid him seeing my side profile and my big nose. But when he saw me, he said I was beautiful without makeup—and I really, really wanted to believe it. His kindness made the voice in my head, the one that kept telling me I was ugly, become a dull whisper. It was a dream come true, like something out of one of my romance novels: nerdy girl gets popular guy, and they fall in love!

Shane was the kind of guy that was the life of the party, so now when we went to those parties, with the same people I had always hung out with, I was no longer the ghost in the room. I still didn't believe I was pretty, but at least I didn't think I was revolting anymore. We did everything together. We had a lot in common. We both loved playing sports, running, and the outdoors. Less than a year later, Shane proposed and I said 'yes'! I was 18 and he was 19. Suddenly people started to pay more attention to me, and Shane's doting on me convinced me that he really did love me. I started to flourish, and I thought that I actually might be happy for the first time in my life.

But life was not without problems. One day, while I was making a turn at a light on my way to high school, someone ran a red light and plowed into my car. I remember having a lot of pain in my neck and feeling dizzy and headachy for quite a while. The doctor gave me a neck brace to wear and looking back, I probably had a mild concussion, but I was young and in love and couldn't be bothered by being tied down with a physical ailment, so I never really took care of it. Instead, I began planning a trip with my friend Janette.

I met my good friend Janette when we were 12, at a German School our parents used to send us to on Saturdays. She lived far away, and it took a couple of years, but our friendship blossomed. As girls, we both dreamed of traveling, promising each other we'd go to Europe when we were 18, and so during my teenage years, I took whatever job I could find to make money for the trip; delivering newspapers, babysitting, teaching swimming, and lifeguarding. While my friends were out buying the latest fashions, I was working and saving money for that plane ticket … but now I had Shane, and while I didn't want to leave my 'schmookie bear', there was no way I was going to give up the dream trip I had worked so hard for.

Shane urged me to go, though he said he'd miss me and was sad we'd be apart for so long. I knew I would miss him too, and so we shortened our trip from two months to just one so that I could be back in his arms once again. Janette agreed to the shorter timeline because she also had a serious boyfriend. We were all set to go that summer after finishing high school.

A week before we were set to leave, I went to the health clinic to get more supply of 'the pill', and when the girl in the office found my chart and opened it, she became very quiet. Suddenly, there was a lot of scurrying around and whispering until finally a manager came and took me to a private room. There, she told me they had tried to reach me and had left me messages (which was not true). Apparently, the pap smear I'd had done many months before showed a high level of abnormal precancerous cells and they needed to do more testing. They asked me to come in the following week, but of course I was going be in Europe and told them I'd make an appointment when I returned.

When I left the office I was a little worried, but by this time I had mastered the art of wearing the mask of 'happy Suzie' and soon I put it out of my mind. Instead, Janette and I got together and … we were *off*. We had an amazing trip, backpacking through Switzerland, Germany, Austria, France, and Italy. We stayed with my cousins in Austria (though not until the end of the trip) and hers in Switzerland, but the rest of the time we stayed in youth hostels. We called home every week, and were pretty responsible considering our age. There were no wild parties or drinking. We met some attractive men along the way, but both Janette and I were completely committed to our own men.

We soon found out that travelling is expensive, and that the money we saved wasn't going quite as far as we hoped, and so we lived on canned Spam and bread, treating ourselves once a week to a fancy restaurant and a glass of wine.

While in the South of France and in Italy, we got hit on by more men than I ever imagined, and my self-confidence began to increase with all the attention. I was feeling very good about myself as we began the last leg of our trip, arriving at my cousins' home in Austria. The next morning, I woke up in the same room I had stayed in as a child … and found I could not open my eyes.

They were completely swollen shut! My cousins took me to the hospital, and the doctor said I had severe allergies. It was strange, because the doctor insisted it was chronic allergies and yet I had never had any allergies at all. We flew home a few days later and Shane met us at the airport. I thought he would take one look and my swollen, red, puffy eyes and run, but he told me he was happy to see me and that I was still beautiful. I never really figured out what caused that allergic reaction.

Once I got home and settled in, life became the same rollercoaster it had always been. For some reason, I had assumed that traveling to foreign places and having adventures would somehow change me. I expected a spark to be ignited in me, a small flame that would make me more confident, or at least more worldly. But that didn't happen. Even with travelling under my belt and a fine young man to love me, there was still something broken inside me.

My health situation did not help. When we returned from Europe, I went back to the health clinic and found that, due to the time lapse while I was travelling, the pre-cancer cells had changed to stage one cervical cancer. I had surgery, it got cleared up ... and I told no one the truth about the diagnosis. I remember Shane and my mom being in the hospital with me, and me telling them that it was no big deal—it was just pre-cancerous cells and not really cancer. I barely remember at all what I was feeling at that time, and I don't remember why I could not tell them the truth. In retrospect, it might be because I did not want to be pitied. I didn't want Shane to look at me differently, and I didn't want my mother to coddle me and over-dramatize things.

When I was a child, and had a simple headache, it would result in my mother saying, "OH YOU POOOOOOR THING! How awwwful!" Her melodic, dread-filled tone as she uttered this always made my skin crawl. She would lose sleep with worry—and would constantly let me know about this great, sleep-depriving worry, which made me feel worse. That day in the hospital, I decided I wasn't a 'poooor thing', it wasn't 'awwwful', and I definitely was not going to be the cause of anyone's lost sleep.

Even as I write this, I realize that I haven't fully unpacked this part of me. To this day, I do not share with my mother the 'bad' things that go on in my life. Though she has toned it down quite a bit, I do not like having to console her over something trivial that has happened to me. It triggers feelings of belittlement and makes me feel that I have to be tough and strong so I don't make her lose sleep.

I started college that September, and started to excel academically. Throughout my earlier schooling, I struggled with my grades, which were only slightly above average. I could not always understand how the teachers taught, and sometimes I felt stupid because things did not make sense. This did not help my low self-esteem and so I found it easier to learn things on my own. In college, this tendency to learn things better on my own was useful. I learned that if I just read the material and figured it out by myself, studying became really easy and much clearer.

Shane and I spent the first year glued to each other's sides, studying together and becoming quite competitive about our marks. With him by my side, I felt that I could accomplish anything ... and I ended up completing my first year with the highest marks in the *entire college*—not just the entire program. I also learned that I had a very high IQ. But those things never felt like much of an accomplishment because it was not my life goal to be a genius. My life goal was to move in with my husband and start a wonderful married life. I'd never really fantasized about what would happen after that. All the movies and books I'd watched and read simply ended with 'happily ever after', so I assumed that after getting married, we would just love each other, have kids, work and be happy. It would be like floating on a bouncy white cloud somewhere close to heaven for the rest of our lives. In retrospect, I clearly understand that those thoughts were pretty simplistic for someone with a near-genius IQ.

But in the meantime I was so happy with Shane that I smothered as much love onto him as I could because my heart was overflowing! I shall highlight the word SMOTHER and the fact that smother and relationships don't go very well together. It felt like I had waited so long to pour out all the love I had bottled up inside, and to bask in his, that I wanted to do absolutely *everything* with him. I didn't want to be apart from him even for a moment. In fact, I even got a job in the same store as him, just so I could be closer to him.

That turned out to be an unexpectedly painful decision. I subsequently found myself getting jealous when I saw other girls talking to him. He was so utterly handsome that women naturally threw themselves at him. He assured me that he only had eyes for me, but doubt crept into my heart. As he started spending time with his friends, I began to fear losing him and I became extremely needy; predictably, as I grew needier, he pulled away—and the more he pulled away, the tighter I held on. Then he announced that his family had to move out of the city, because they could not afford to stay, and my fear of losing him escalated. As my neediness grew, he pulled away even more.

I cannot really blame him for cheating on me. But when I found out, my world as I knew it came to an end. We were just about to go into the second year of paramedic school together, and now I would have to see him every single day with his new girlfriend—one of our classmates.

The first thing that came into my head after I found out he had chosen another woman over me was that I was not good enough, and I would never be good enough, for anyone. I thought about ending my life again, but decided not to. Instead, I made a vow to myself that I would never let myself love anyone so deeply ever again. I repeated this mantra every day. It was so deep and solemn that it would stick with me for almost 20 years. Never again would I let my heart be that vulnerable or trusting. I spent a few days in my bed crying but then I buried myself in work and studying so that I did not have to deal with the wrenching pain in my heart.

This vow of mine did not stop my yearning to be part of a 'we', however. Within a month I began searching phone ads trying to find someone to fill the void Shane's betrayal had left. At that time there was no internet, so dating was done by responding to newspaper ads, and arranging dates via phone. When asked about my past relationship, I usually pushed aside the fact that I had been needy and clingy; instead, I wore the badge of an innocent victim when I told the tale.

In my mind, I had been the perfect doting girlfriend and he was the creep that cheated.

Jeff

I've always had problems with my knees, even when I was a kid in elementary school. My kneecaps would just sporadically pop out of place, which caused me a lot of pain. One day while I was playing college volleyball I went up for a spike and, upon landing, 'pop' went my knee. I was wearing one of those braces with the hole around the kneecap, but somehow my kneecap found a way to move all the way over and out anyway. I smacked it back into place, but the pain was too much, and my leg swelled up like a balloon.

Shane, my now ex-fiancé, happened to be there and he offered to take me to the hospital. I am not sure why I let him take me. I think I was hoping that he would realize how wrong he had been and come back to me, but more likely he just felt bad for having cheated and was being kind. Of course he just dumped me, and my reconciliation fantasy, at the emergency room doors and sped off, leaving me alone to hobble into the emergency room. Understandably, the hurt in my heart was greater than the one in my knee. I felt like a fool for thinking he would come back to me.

At the hospital, the doctors put my leg in a brace and ordered an arthroscopic surgery, which I went through like a zombie. The surgeon said that they were not sure what was causing my knee problems, but that I had hypermobile kneecaps and some tearing that they cleaned up. He then told me that the pain and symptoms I was experiencing did not match up to what they thought the problem was, so they sent me to physiotherapy. The physiotherapy helped and my knee healed fairly quickly after that, though it would still dislocate from time to time.

When I felt better, I tried 'personals' dating again and soon met Jeff on a phone dating site. His sexy European accent reminded me of Tomas and drew me in right away. After a series of phone calls, we decided to meet in person. Jeff was a few years older than I was, had a decent job and was ready to move out on his own. He had a rugged handsomeness to him, curly brown hair and green eyes. Jeff was really sweet, a little quiet and shy, and obviously taken by me, though I can't say I would have been attracted if I had met him randomly. However, his attraction to me was enough, and we got serious fast. I was happy again because someone adored me! Those voices telling me how unlovable I was were wrong!

Jeff was doting and romantic. He, too, had been hurt in a previous relationship, and this drew us closer together. After four months of dating, he took me to a fancy restaurant, got down on one knee, and proposed. I said 'yes'.

I was over the moon at this turn of events, but very soon after we got engaged, Jeff started getting possessive and controlling. One night we went out to a club with a few other couples and soon the girls and I were out on the dance floor, leaving the guys chatting with their beers in hand. To me this was normal behavior, so I was quite surprised when, on the ride home, Jeff got angry with me and yelled, "You just left me standing like a spare dick while you danced!"

I was shocked by this reaction. Shane had *never* yelled at me. I felt panic rise in my chest and I couldn't breathe as my heart raced. "But I was just dancing with the *girls*!" I argued in defense.

This only seemed to fuel his anger. He accused me of trying to attract other men while he had to sit and watch. I had trouble processing what he was saying. I'd never thought about attracting other men—I hadn't even wanted to dance, but the girls had asked me to. We kept arguing until something inside of me backed down. I apologized, he calmed down and then he told me he loved me so much that he couldn't stand the thought of other men wanting me and looking at me, while inside my head I was thinking, *who would want to look at me anyway?* The next day he apologized and bought me flowers.

There was no way I could handle another breakup, so I pushed down the red flags that were waving frantically inside my head and we carried on. I believed him when he told me that everything would be fine once we were married, and that he was just nervous about the wedding. I did not acknowledge that the reason I carried on was because of the belief deep inside me that if I didn't marry him, no one else would ever want me. Besides, I had just emptied my savings to buy a condo, and we were about to move in. The condo was an absolutely stunning lower penthouse, with floor to ceiling windows overlooking a forest, in an up-and-coming posh neighborhood. The whole notion of marrying a European man with a stable job and beautiful new home seemed outwardly like one of my romance novels. There was no turning back! We were married a month after I graduated as a paramedic.

The wedding was a grandiose affair, straight out of a fairytale. It was literally what every girl dreams of, with the elegant ballroom, dinner and dancing, and my princess gown. Just for a moment, I was a star and people were fawning over me. It was riveting.

I invited as many of my old school friends as I could, as if to prove that I wasn't such a loser after all, and that this ugly duckling *could* marry a handsome prince. Just before the ceremony, a friend asked if I was sure that this was what I wanted to do. Even though there was a little voice inside me that knew something was wrong, my desire to have a husband and a 'happily ever after' had long overtaken it. "Absolutely," I said with a smile.

Jeff had some erectile dysfunction, which he put down to being a psychological result of having been cheated on. I knew this before we got married, but I thought it would go away with time as his confidence grew. It did get a little better, but his insecurity fed my insecurity, and our honeymoon was a disaster. One day we were lying on the cruise ship deck sunning ourselves and some people invited us to play volleyball. He didn't want to go, but I was very excited to play again, so I went. After the game was over Jeff became enraged, accusing me of trying to flirt with other guys. I hadn't spoken to, or even *looked* at anyone! Still, he was very jealous. We didn't speak for three days, as I refused to apologize. We arrived home and I told everyone what an amazing honeymoon we'd had, and we never spoke of it again.

But things started to get worse in our marriage. After that, Jeff became controlling of my every move. He would yell, scream and belittle me for not putting the cap back on the toothpaste, or not putting my shoes in the closet. Soon, we stopped having sex completely. Me being me, internally I took the blame. I assumed his erection problem was because I was not good enough or pretty enough and, thinking I could solve the problem by becoming a better wife, I began making his lunches and dinners and took care of all the housework. He never helped.

In those days it was hard to get a full-time job as a paramedic, so I had several part-time jobs instead. I worked with the city, had another job with a medical company that provided emergency support at professional sporting events, and I also did patient transfers. I loved what I did wholeheartedly, and would work long hours. However this, combined with my perceived responsibility for housework and keeping my husband happy, wore me out. Only four months into my marriage I was miserable and I felt like a slave. Jeff and I barely spoke and, when we did, there was unbearable tension. I felt trapped and alone living with him in a city away from everyone I knew.

I was still friends with Jannette, and she and her husband came over for dinner once. Afterward, she called me to say she was a little concerned that I was doing everything while Jeff just sat there expecting to be served. I told her we took turns playing host, and that everything was okay. But it was a lie. I did not want anyone to know how lonely I felt in the marriage.

At work, I was regularly partnered with Earl. Earl made me laugh so much, which was something I had not done in quite a while. He was really easy to talk to and, during our long 12-hour shifts, I began opening up to him about what was going on in my marriage and how I knew I had made a mistake in marrying Jeff. He was so sympathetic and comforting that I couldn't help having feelings for him. I was emotionally cheating on my husband—although I justified it by convincing myself that Jeff didn't care about me. I loved the attention and thought a little innocent flirting could not harm anyone. One day Earl told me he was in love with me, and I suddenly wished I was single. He made me feel pretty and desired where Jeff no longer did.

Meanwhile, at home Jeff was becoming more and more abusive. He would push me and accuse me of cheating. He would yell at me and call me names. When it started, I had not even met Earl yet and *wasn't* cheating, although after meeting Earl, I certainly entertained the idea. Friends and family thought Jeff and I were so happy because, of course, I had to be true to the mask everyone saw and knew. I could not let anyone know what was really going on because I was filled with regret and shame. I was angry at myself for not listening to the voice inside me that had questioned my decision to marry Jeff. I was scared at the thought of being a failure. But I had also gotten so good at pretending things were okay that I didn't even know what I wanted anymore. I felt like a feather floating in the breeze.

I began to resist Jeff and his control. He had obsessive-compulsive disorder (OCD) and occasionally, I would get revenge by deliberately leaving the house in a mess. I would purposely leave my shoes out of the closet, or my coat slung over the couch, just to make him crazy. After all, who was he to think he could boss me around?

Admittedly, I'm not proud of such behavior today, but then again, I was only 22 and the frontal lobe of my brain had not fully developed. Further, I was confused and angry because my marriage was not at all like the romance novels I had read. There was nothing simple about the relationship, and there was no 'happily ever after' in sight. Jeff stopped being nice to me and seemed to expect me to be 'the little wife' who would cook and clean for him. Never mind my 12-to-14-hour shifts; he would come home from work and wait for things to be done while he put his feet up.

This didn't sit well with me at all. I did not want to play 'Suzie homemaker' anymore, nor did I want to be a slave to this emotionally abusive man. My house was not a home, and I started getting a sinking feeling in my stomach every time I walked through our condo doors. Talking on the phone with friends was my only outlet, but it made him insecure. He would ask who I was talking to, and why I was talking, and then would sit and listen to my conversations. When I was done, he would say that obviously he was not enough for me if I needed to talk to other people so much.

During the 1990s, female paramedics were rare, which meant I was generally paired with men when I was on shift. Naturally, after being in a cab with someone for over 12 hours, I began to develop friendships with my male colleagues and talk more openly about my life than people in other work situations might do. Also, the nature of the job is that you spend your day experiencing trauma with your colleagues, which lends itself to a type of intimacy that is deeper than your average work connection. I grew close to the people I worked with, and sometimes shared crude jokes with them as part of our work banter.

Jeff did not like that I worked with male partners; he wanted me to get into real estate with his father. He was very threatened by these close relationships to the point that, on one occasion, he dragged me out of my work Christmas party, enraged at what he described as my 'flirtatious' behavior while talking with my co-workers.

Jeff's face was red with anger as he sped home, yelling and screaming at me the whole way. I was scared. When we got up to our condo the fight escalated, his accusations and my defenses flying in a heated exchange. It ended up with him hitting me in the face. Shocked and frightened, I immediately retreated to the bathroom, where I locked myself in for the night. Jeff went to bed, while I crawled into the bathtub and cried myself to sleep.

The next morning, I walked into the kitchen to find flowers and a teary-eyed Jeff, apologizing and promising that he would never do that again. He expected me to rush to him with open arms, but I just couldn't. He had been verbally abusive to me for so many months that I was upset and confused about what to do. The thought of leaving the marriage terrified me … but so did the thought of staying.

We decided to go for coffee to talk about it. Another fight ensued in the car and he became furious. He screeched to a halt at the side of the road in a remote area, leaned over and opened my car door, unbuckled my seatbelt, pushed me out of the car, and then sped off. I had no money and was far from home. It was winter and there was a deep blanket of snow everywhere. My hair that was still wet from my morning shower. I was terrified. I knew I had to leave him, but my parents had not even finished paying off the wedding bill off. His parents owed my parents a lot of money as they had agreed to pay for half the wedding, that at the time they could not afford to. My parents had agreed to loan them $6000 which remained outstanding. How could I leave? How could I stay? My parents would never get their money back.

Trembling in fear and shivering from the cold as ice formed on my wet hair, I began walking. I was in a bewildered daze, not really believing what had just transpired. I made it to a store where I called a friend. He told me to call the police. I had a bruise on my face from the night before, proving that he'd hit me, so that is exactly what I did.

The police picked me up and took me back home. We found Jeff eating breakfast as if nothing had happened. Just the sight of him, sitting there calmly at the table with his eggs and toast, caused such a feeling of anger to well up inside me that my heart almost exploded. He had not even come looking for me! How was this love? I had been gone three hours in the dead of winter with no money and no phone while he cooked up a feast for himself. I decided then and there to tell the police everything. They took pictures of my face. They took pictures of the fresh tire marks going into our parking garage from when Jeff had driven like a maniac the night before. They arrested him and took him to jail.

I had never been more terrified in my life. Here I was, 22 years old, living far from away all of my friends and family, and my husband of five months was now in jail for assaulting me. I couldn't tell my parents. I couldn't tell anyone. What would they think? I felt like a complete failure. How would I explain this to people? This would confirm that I truly was an unlovable loser. All I had wanted was to be happy and have love, and it was crushing my very soul to realize there was no such thing as a happy ending. By this time, I was so self-involved with my own victimhood that those ominous dark voices wanting me to end my life, had dulled. What replaced them was anger and determination.

Jeff's parents called me a few days later to try to convince me to drop the charges. Jeff was now staying with them and wanted to see me. I refused. I didn't know what to do. I ran into Earl's arms and cried while he wiped away my tears with kisses. *If Earl loves me*, I thought, *maybe I am still worthy.* I felt shame that I could not hold a marriage down more than five months. I felt guilty Jeff's parents owed my parents so much money. I didn't know what to do, and finally I got to the point where I could not say no when his parents kept calling (I later learned in therapy that I could not really say no to anybody, for fear of disapproval). Ultimately, I agreed to talk to my husband.

Jeff cried on the phone and said he knew he was wrong and that he loved me and wanted to keep our marriage. I told him I would think about it. I may have even led him to believe that there was still a slight chance that I was going to forgive him because, as I've mentioned, I was afraid to say 'no'. I stalled by telling him I needed some time ... but what I really needed was time to myself to figure things out and to get the courage to leave. However, I just couldn't do it—because my worst fear was being alone and unloved.

Meanwhile, my affection for kind, sweet Earl grew until one day during a moment of bad judgement, I brought Earl back to the condo on our break. Somehow Jeff found out I was home, pulled up and saw someone else's car in my parking spot. Jeff literally broke the door down while Earl and I were in bed.

My heart had never pounded so fast. I was filled with sheer terror. I don't even know why I got into bed with Earl except, perhaps, to prove to myself that I was still desirable. Thankfully, Earl was a pretty big guy, and Jeff took off. Earl left, and I was a wreck. I had to go back to work and I shook my entire shift. It was a relief that there were no serious calls that night and I was able to keep it together. I was partnered with a different paramedic that shift, and I told him I had a stomachache to explain my anxious, distracted behavior. I got home around midnight that night to find a message on my answering machine from my mother. "Suzie," she said, "Jeff is here and told us everything that you did. We know what you have done and that you have been cheating on him. You are no longer our daughter, and you are not to contact us again."

There are no words that can describe how that knife in my heart felt. Remnants of it stayed for years. How could my parents, who were supposed to love me, just throw me out of their lives with such ease? Was I that worthless? Did they ever even care for me at all? I felt so shocked, alone, and defeated. I didn't care anymore about the money. My marriage was over. My friends were 50 kilometers away and now I no longer had parents. I couldn't even tell my friends because of the shame I felt. How could my parents just disown me without even hearing my side? I was their daughter! But it seemed so easy for them to just shut me out of their life. How could that possibly be love? Again, the conflict arose between feeling completely worthless or just pulling up my sleeves and carrying on as my soul was being torn in two.

I pushed my emotions aside and buried myself in Earl. Like a robot, I was just going through the motions of things that had to be done. I didn't allow myself to feel guilty about Earl. I packed up and sold the condo. Jeff's father was a real estate agent and they swindled me out of all my savings, but I didn't care. I found out that during our brief marriage, Jeff had secretly taken my savings out of my bank account to lend to his parents, so I really had nothing. At that point, I had no fight left in me so I let it go. Earl was the only person in my life who was feeding my soul, and I clung to him as a kind of lifeline. He helped me find a little bachelor apartment in the west end of the city. It was tiny, and not in the best neighbourhood, but it was all I could afford. I was finally free of Jeff and his family.

It is funny how life works to give you a dose of your own medicine. When I was obsessed and clingy with Shane, I could not understand why he didn't want all this love I had to pour out. Well, I got to be on the other end of the stick with Earl. As I was gaining strength, working more, and finally facing my friends, he got more and more smothering. At first, I liked the attention. He never wanted to leave my side and would even follow me to the bathroom. He was continually asking me how I was feeling and was never satisfied with the answer because he wanted me to go deeper. "But how are you REALLY feeling?" he would ask. He could talk about our feelings for days.

Perhaps he was trying to break down my walls, or get the clingy, desperate girl I'd been when we met back. Whatever it was, I eventually began to get irritated by his incessant doting and started feeling like a pet in a cage. He always had his hands on me and would get wounded when I wasn't affectionate back. He would cry endlessly if I didn't tell him I loved him every hour we were together.

I had to break up with him, but I couldn't find the words. I didn't want to hurt Earl or have him hate me. I gathered the courage to tell him that I needed some time apart from him. I may have left him with a shred of hope that a future was possible because I couldn't say no when he begged me to reconsider.

George

Two weeks later, I went to the Dominican Republic with Margaret, a high school acquaintance with whom I had recently reconnected. She was single and alone, and had just been through a breakup too. We made a spur of the moment decision that we both needed a vacation and so we bought tickets and away we went.

When we arrived, we enjoyed the warm climate, drank copious amounts of alcohol, and at night got all dolled up in revealing clothes and went dancing. It was on one of these magical nights that I met George, a fellow Canadian.

George approached me at a nightclub, and while I wasn't particularly interested in him, he was very interested in me. He kept working on me; he had a good sense of humor, a nice smile, and told me I was the most beautiful woman he had ever laid eyes on. Of course I loved the attention, and by now you recognize my pattern. I became interested because he was interested in me.

As I got to know George, I saw how well put together he was and decided that that was just what I needed in my life. He was a few years older than me, had a successful career as a top financial advisor in a major bank, had plenty of friends, and played hockey on the weekends. He was decent looking but what attracted me to him was his easy-going nature. Most importantly, he was not smothering.

Because he lived relatively near me, when we got back from vacation we started dating. I hadn't heard from Earl and I felt relieved, and hoped he had moved on. I have to say, out of all the men I have ever been with, George was by far the most normal and kind-hearted.

A month or so after we began dating, George and I and a group of friends went up to George's cottage, which was on a small lake nestled deep in a thick forest, the nearest town 30 minutes away. It was winter and there was so much snow we had to use snowmobiles to gain get there. The purpose of these weekend jaunts, I soon discovered, was to drink and pretend to be ice fishing.

The next day, we took the snowmobiles out and George let me drive. I had never been on one before, and it was thrilling to speed through the forest. I was finally starting to feel at peace, and while the icy wind bit at my face, I felt a stirring in my heart. George's life seemed exciting, filled with adventure and stable. It was alluring. I thought to myself, *maybe I can let myself love him.*

When we arrived back at the cottage, I was filled with a brighter spirit and just wanted to rush over to George and kiss him. However, as I swung my leg over the snowmobile to get off, I heard a loud snap in my knee, which was followed by intense pain—and suddenly I was on the ground. This time I knew whatever had happened to my knee was worse than all the other times. Someone watching said that they saw my body go one way and my leg go the other. It was obvious I had to be taken to the hospital.

I dimly remember being strapped to a sled for a long bumpy ride behind a snowmobile back to our cars. The hospitals up in cottage country are not exactly renowned for specialized care, so we decided to make the three-hour trek back to the city.

The surgeon at the hospital told me there was extensive damage. He even called in a few residents to show them my knees, saying he had never seen anyone with such hypermobile kneecaps, or such rare symptoms. I was put in a splint and told I would need major reconstructive surgery, but they had to wait for things to settle down before they could do it. The doctor also told me the surgery would have me incapacitated for at least three months, and that I would have to stay in bed. He recommended that I have someone home with me as I would need a lot of care once I was discharged from the hospital.

This presented a very big problem for me, because I had still not spoken to my parents so I couldn't go there. George still lived with his parents, and our relationship was new, so having him look after me was not an option either. Worse, it was impossible to stay in my apartment as there were stairs to climb that I would not be able to navigate—and even if I could, I would not be able to afford my rent since I would be off work.

Still hurt by what my parents had said to me, I had no intention of calling them … but as the days went on, I realized there really were no other options. I had no other family I could lean on, and none of my friends could help me. The only option was to make the call to my parents, tail between my legs—but I just couldn't do it. I was still hurt and angry at them for not even listening to my side of the story, and so casually tossing me out of their lives.

A couple of weeks later I was still in my apartment, waiting to recover enough to have the surgery. My apartment was a tiny, one-room bachelor, and I was alone. After a week, I was ready to crawl out of my skin with boredom.

One day, I was lying in bed staring up at my ceiling, wracking my brain as I tried to figure out how to talk to my parents, when Earl barged in. My heart leapt up into my throat. I had forgotten to lock my doors, and he was angry that I hadn't called him when I got back from my trip. He said he wanted me back, and that I'd had enough time to think about our relationship.

Shocked, I got up and tried to hobble away on my crutches, but he grabbed them from me and also tore the phone cord out of my wall. I was in shock, and had no idea what to do. I stared at this man who had once been so jovial and sweet, and who I now barely recognized. His once handsome face was contorted into a scowl. In a shaking voice, I stammered out that he was a great guy, that I cared about him, but I was seeing someone else now, and we were not meant to be together.

He collapsed on the ground in tears, saying that I was his soul mate as he asked me how I could do this to him. It took three hours to talk him down, and the whole time I was shaking inside. I reminded him of all his good qualities, and told him that there was someone out there for him who could give him everything I could not. Eventually he left. I was relieved, but cried myself to sleep.

The visit from Earl was the tipping point that fueled my desire to get as far away from that end of the city, and Earl, as I could. Pushing all of my emotions aside, I decided to call my parents and ask for help. I swallowed my pride, took a deep breath, and dialed their number. My mother's voice became cold when she realized it was me on the phone. I told her I was sorry for what had happened, but that I had an accident and needed surgery. She briskly replied that she was sorry to hear about my knee and would talk to my father.

A week later, my father met me in a mall coffee shop. I was still in a cast and on crutches, so getting there was not exactly easy. He said I could come back and live with them but there were 'conditions' to me being allowed back in their life. He said they did not want to know what happened in my marriage, but what I had done was wrong and I was never to speak about it. My dad then told me that I was a 'virago woman' and I had always been a heathen. I had no idea what a virago woman meant, but it did not sound good. I was not in a position to ask about it, so I held my tongue.

I sat silently with my casted leg up on a chair swallowing back my tears. Dad must have noticed my eyes get watery, because his expression softened and he said that no matter what, they loved me and would help. If I was to live under their roof, however, I would have to be home at a reasonable hour, let them know where I was—and under no circumstance would I be allowed to have any boyfriends around them again. As we stood up to go, he gave me an awkward hug and said he was sorry about my knee. There was no offer to help me move, just a request to let them know in advance when I would be arriving so they could have the room arranged.

When I got home, my leg was throbbing, but I couldn't find the tears I wanted to cry so I grabbed my dictionary to find out what a 'virago woman' was. I found two definitions: A virago woman could be either a loud, overbearing, manly woman or a warrior-type woman with great strength and courage. I was pretty sure he meant the first one, because the tone in his voice was not indicative of a compliment. In fact, he went on to call me this several times over the next ten years, each time with a frown on his face. Once I asked him what it meant. He muttered something about being a stubborn type of woman who wasn't very womanly; what he did not realize was that upon learning the meaning of 'virago woman', the tiniest seed was planted inside of me which years later would sprout into a drive to become a warrior. Yet that day, as I sat on my fancy European couch in my small crappy apartment, the word still hurt. As always, I buried that pain.

George was very understanding about me moving in with my parents, but I could not tell him the whole truth about why he could not come and visit me there. I just said my parents weren't ready to meet anyone new. A few weeks later, my brother Nick and my friend Margaret came to the rescue and helped me pack up and move. Nick had already helped me move the last two times, and he never asked me any questions about why I was moving; instead, he just rolled up his sleeves and dug in.

A few months later, I wound up telling him the truth about my marriage. His first reaction was that he wanted to find Jeff and beat the crap out of him—and he was furious at my parents.

We bonded over this and then we talked a little about how strict our parents were. Nick recalled a time when my dad kicked him in the back and sent him flying across the hall. I remembered the incident. We had had a large neighborhood barbeque in our backyard, and all the kids started to have a food fight. My dad had caught Nick tossing a piece of bread at his friend and yelled at us both to get in the house. I don't remember exactly what happened, but there was a lot of yelling and objects being thrown. I remembered sitting on my bedroom listening to Nick cry, and crying along with him, as my dad screamed at him. I was scared … because I knew my turn was next. And then the memory faded to black.

Nick and I both agreed the incident was pretty messed up, and laughed nervously as we talked about it. We didn't know how to deal with our feelings, and so Nick lit up a joint, cracked a few jokes and it was soon forgotten. We never discussed it again, because neither of us really knew how to talk to each other. In retrospect, I wish we'd known how, and been able to express how we felt and how the wounds of our childhood had created scarred adults; I wish we'd been able to say how mean our parents were and how we never felt loved. Maybe if we had been able to open up, it would have saved so much heartache in our futures. We didn't. We did what we knew best, which was to bury our hurt and put on a smile.

The reconstructive surgery went well but I needed three surgeries in total on that knee. They cut the bone in half, moved and repositioned it and screwed it back in place, and they reconstructed a tendon. I was in a cast from my ankle to my hip for over three months. I was told to stay in bed for six weeks, but after three weeks, I started getting antsy to be out of my parent's house. The energy in there was so thick and heavy. My parents were helpful, but there was a cold detachment to their care. I needed to get out of there.

I taught myself to drive with my left foot, propping up my casted leg on the passenger seat. Just before the knee incident, I had gotten a supplementary job, part-time temporary office work, and so I went back to that. I was determined to get back to living on my own as soon as possible, but with my injury, working as a paramedic would be hard, if possible at all. I had to think about what I would do with my life if I couldn't be a paramedic, though I was not ready to give up on a job I loved.

When the cast came off, I was somewhat shocked to see this hairy stick of a leg with a large scar on it that belonged to me. The negative voice in my head tried to tell me how this scar would make me uglier and more unattractive than ever, but George encouraged me not to think that way.

At home, my parents were slowly starting to be a little warmer to me, and even met George briefly, although they kept him at arm's length. I think they felt sorry for me and saw I was determined to persevere. I worked hard in physiotherapy to get my physical abilities back, and eventually I went back to jogging and then to my paramedic work. It felt good to put on my uniform again and help people. It made me feel like I had a purpose in life. I have to admit, I also enjoyed getting male attention when I wore my uniform. It soothed my deep insecurity to have men look at me, whistle or say, "Help, I need mouth to mouth!" It was corny, but it made me smile. Suzie was back!

Two months later, disaster struck again when I hurt my back on the job, sustaining a second-degree tear in one of my muscles. Worse, since I was only working part-time, in a contract position, I had no benefits. After rehab, I tried to return to my job but it was clear that I would not be able to sustain heavy lifting. This was basically the end of my career, which was hard for me to accept. Being a paramedic was all I ever wanted to do (outside of being the star of my own romance novel). It gave me purpose; if I couldn't heal the emptiness inside me, at least I could help others. I felt so lost and unsure of what to do with my life. My schooling had been so specific and tailored that there were not really any other options than to work at that job.

George and I were still together but I felt confused about what direction to go with my life. Finally, I decided to go backpacking in Europe with my friend Margaret for the summer, hoping as I had so long ago on my trip with Jannette to find answers and 'discover myself'.

George was very understanding about my decision and so Margaret and I flew to Europe and proceeded to have a fabulous time. We went paragliding and white water rafting in Switzerland, drank at pubs in London, smoked exotic weed in Amsterdam, ate paella and drank Sangria in Spain, sunbathed in Nice, France, toured Italy and drank ouzo and partied hard in Greece. We stayed in youth hostels or slept on trains. We met so many people, and sometimes we would meet the same ones quite randomly in a completely different country weeks later. There was a very attractive guy who liked me, and I was very tempted to be with him, but in the end, I didn't.

Towards the end of our trip, while we were in Greece, we decided to purchase a plane ticket from a travel agency in Corfu to fly from Athens to London. Originally, we were supposed to take the train back, but we were tired and wanted to spend more time roaming the Greek Islands. We spent the last week drinking a lot of alcohol and eating so many gyros and baklava that my clothes were getting tight.

On our last day in Greece, a few hours before take-off, we hailed a cab and gave him the address on our plane ticket. The taxi pulled into an old, abandoned airfield, and we were confused. We did not speak Greek and he spoke no English so, thinking there must have been some kind of mix-up, we told him to take us to the airport. We arrived early and spent the last of our money in a shop before lining up to get our boarding passes.

We were in a very long lineup in a small room with no air conditioning, and we were carrying 40-pound backpacks. When it was our turn to board, we produced our tickets—and were told by the lady at the counter that our tickets were not valid. We stared at her in bewilderment as it sank in that we had been sold fraudulent tickets. Frantic, we asked what flights were available, because had a connecting flight from London back home the next evening, and I was to start work two days after that. We were told there were no tickets available at all for another two weeks with their airline, and that no other airlines were selling tickets either. She told us our only option was to try to fly standby.

Defeated, we sat down and listened to many others talking about how they had been stranded in the country for days. We hadn't realized how busy the last two weeks in August are in Europe. We'd also maxed out our credit cards, so even if we got lucky and found a flight, we had no way to pay for it. I tried calling home but could not reach my parents. Nick answered the phone and was completely stoned and just laughed. So I called George. He wired money into my bank account and we felt a little less hopeless.

As night fell and all the airport kiosks closed, we lined up in the standby line. The booths would not reopen until six the next morning, and there were two girls in front of us. Around midnight Margaret, exhausted by the sweltering heat, decided to go and lie down outside the airport doors. I refused to give up our spot in line. I stayed as the line behind us grew slowly throughout the night. I prayed and asked God to find us a way home.

About an hour after the booths re-opened the next morning, it was announced that there were two available seats left on the flight we wanted. Our hearts sank because the two girls in front of us would be the ones flying home; however, as they got to the counter, one girl could not find her passport, and so they could not take the seats. We were so relieved when we got on that plane.

By that time, having stayed up all night partying the night prior, I had been awake for 48 hours. I was okay with it because I thought I could just sleep on the plane, but I was wrong. I tried to sleep, but back then they allowed people to smoke inside the planes and it was stuffy, smoky and horrible, and so sleep never came.

Luckily, when we got to London we were able to catch our flight home, but by then I was so wound up with adrenaline that I could not sleep on that flight either. By the time we got home, I had been awake for 72 hours straight. Being awake that long can cause hallucinations and I was not immune! The walls looked like they were swaying in a breeze, and when I met George at the airport I called him Shane and began mumbling to myself. George took me home and I slept for two days straight.

Juan

The funny thing about unresolved, suppressed emotional issues is that they are always waiting for you when you get home. One can never run far or long enough. Once again, I thought I would have some sort of epiphany about the meaning of life, and the direction I was supposed to take, when I got home from my trip, but it never came.

With my paramedic career in tatters, I decided to go back to school to study nursing, but that only lasted one year. I wanted to be an emergency room nurse, but that meant I'd need another three years of education, and I was not patient enough. In the back of my mind, I was still hoping for my fantasy life the house, white picket fence, husband, and 2.2 children. Giving up on nursing, I found a job in the claims department of an insurance agency. It paid decently and was interesting, and I planned to be there only for one year.

I was still living at my parents' home, and it was making me antsy. My brother had moved to the other side of the country a few months prior, so I decided to visit him. We spent a week exploring the city he lived in and smoking pot. Marijuana wasn't really my thing, but he loved it. Since our teens, we had been quite disconnected, and I wanted to change that. At first, it was a little awkward because we didn't really know each other as adults.

Over the years, I'd been busy with boyfriends and he'd been very much into experimenting with drugs, so we'd never had any real conversations. We did not have much in common anymore, so I broke the ice by getting high with him ... and soon we began to grow closer again.

I decided when I returned home that it was time to move out of my parents' house. I found an apartment and got a roommate, who was the girlfriend of one of my dance partners. I had started salsa dancing and, because of my dance background, I caught on very quickly.

As I made these important steps in an effort to move forward in my life, I started to become unhappy with my relationship. George and I had been together for about two years by then, yet I still felt lost inside. In my brokenness, I convinced myself that I was bored with George and that a future with him would be boring. In reality, my feelings were partly because I could not accept that I deserved to have someone so stable and well put together, but also because George lacked some emotional depth and spirituality. He was genuinely nice and caring, but he was a 30-year-old man with a high-paying job who still lived at home with his parents and was catered to by his mother. She packed his lunches and ironed his shirts every single day. I didn't want to be the one to fill that role if we ever moved in together; I had been that kind of wife to Jeff—and there was no way I was going to do it again. I really hurt him when I broke it off with him, and I regret that. He really was a nice guy.

Single for the first time in a while, I worked and I danced. Soon I got an evening job at a dance studio, and I loved it. I went salsa dancing most nights, sometimes as many as five nights a week. Being on the dance floor with the beat of the drums pounding in my chest made me feel free and happy, if only for those moments.

But, as always, there was a battle going on inside me. I was desperate for someone to love me and treat me well—because

I knew what kind of treatment I *didn't* want—but at the same time I subconsciously craved a 'bad guy'. I wondered if there was something wrong with me for feeling this way, but I quickly shoved these doubts aside and bounced back quickly into the dating scene. Along the way, I had surgery on my foot for a bunion, and I had a deviated septum repaired in my nose. During nose surgery, I had them reduce the size a bit, as I was still convinced my nose was too big and I was still a little anxious about letting people see my profile. This turned out to be a big mistake because after the surgery, while I could breathe better, I developed a lot of scar tissue in my nose, which made it look like a bulb. Insecurity flooded over me again; I hated the way I looked and I had to have another surgery a year later to fix it.

Somewhere between these surgeries I met Juan at a salsa club. I would go salsa dancing at these clubs in my skimpy outfits, believing that the only thing about me that would ever attract a man was my body. Despite the fact that I had a small chest, the rest of me was toned and the gangly limbs I'd had as a teenager were lean and strong.

Juan was tall, dark, handsome, emotionally unavailable, and perfect for me. He was very tall with dark tanned latin skin, very fit, and very handsome. He was always impeccably dressed in suit and tie and behaved like such a gentleman. He liked to have fun, and that was just what I thought I needed. He told me right off the bat that he would be an eternal bachelor and that he never wanted to settle down. Subconsciously, something in me saw that as a challenge. I would win his love! And so I set about trying to become the perfect girlfriend. He encouraged me to get a breast enhancement and so I did, to please him. I'd noticed he always stared at women with large breasts, and I'd never liked mine, so I thought, *why not?*

Juan liked well-styled, glamorous women with fine manners, so I started layering on the make-up and dressing like a barbie doll.

I thought it would make him look at me more than at the other girls in the salsa clubs we went to. I thought I was in love.

A few months into our relationship, Juan told me that he was going to get deported and that he was looking for someone to pay so he could get married and get his papers to stay in the country. Panic filled me. What if he fell in love with this new 'wife'? I couldn't have my 'Prince Charming' marry someone else, so I offered to marry him until he gained his citizenship and then divorce him after that. We got married. My parents didn't even know.

At the ceremony, he had arranged to have a song played that was my favorite and had become 'our' song. This led me to believe that I had a chance of getting *real* love from Juan, and that our marriage was more than just a fake wedding. He was doting and I became more and more convinced that he had feelings for me. While I was used to creating staged pictures of our happy 'married' life to fool immigration, Juan went one step further, setting up his apartment with rose petals, champagne, and candles for me when there wasn't anyone there to take any more pictures. I was more enthused about him than ever after that.

However, things changed the very next day when he said he had plans for the day. Confused, I went home to my apartment, wondering why had he gone through so much romantic effort the night before, just to send me off the next day with a cold 'thank-you'. In my fantasy land, Juan was supposed to fall madly in love with me and not want a divorce, and we'd live happily ever after.

I remained willfully blind. Even finding a woman's underwear in his jacket pocket one day a couple of months later was not enough for me to give up my dream. Finally a woman called me one day. She told me she had seen us together and realized that Juan wasn't single, as she had thought. She told me he had been hitting on her, provocatively touching her, and had tried to kiss her a few days prior. They had even been out together a few times, but she hadn't known he had a girlfriend. I told her I was not his girlfriend; I was his wife! She apologized profusely and then said she was a Christian, and that was why she wanted me to know the truth.

I did not really understand what she meant in saying she was a Christian. I had been brought up in Catholic school, though, so I told her I was a Christian too. She was so apologetic and kind, and she told me she would not talk to him anymore. Juan, of course, denied everything and said they were just friends. He said he never tried to kiss her, and she must have gotten the wrong idea. My gut told me he was lying, but there was no way I could face another breakup. I was so incredibly hurt, and told him I needed some time to think.

Enter the steep drop downward on my rollercoaster as the black cloud that had loomed over me throughout my childhood and youth, returned with a vengeance. I spiraled into silent deep depression all within a few days, but I hid it well. Not even my roommate knew what I was going through, because on the exterior I was all smiles and laughs. However, inside I was sad and confused and without hope.

On the third night after this plummet into emotional hell, while alone in my apartment, a feeling of desperation overwhelmed me. I felt I could not go on living, because I really was unlovable. Here I was, fake married and clinging to a fantasy that my fake husband would grow to love me, but he had cheated on me. How could anyone love me? There was nothing of me to love—or so the voice in my head kept telling me. I totally believed that no one would even notice if I was not around anymore, and I truly believed that life was not worth living if I had to be alone.

My roommate was out of town for the week, and so I did not have to hide what I was doing. It was if something had overtaken my body and all awareness of my surroundings had been taken away. All I could think about was that I had to end my life. I methodically and carefully counted out 40 narcotic pills that I had left over from various surgeries, swallowed them one by one, and went to bed. There was no emotion in me as I swallowed those pills. It was as if I was on auto-pilot, completely detached from what was happening. I felt no sadness, only emptiness—and focus on the task at hand. I just knew I didn't want to suffer anymore.

As a paramedic, I knew which pills would do the trick. I was convinced it would work and my pain would end. I did not even leave a note for anyone. I have heard people talk about the kind of agony a person must go through before ending their life, and how awful it must be. It was not that way for me. It was so cold and calculated that it felt as if I was already dead before I even opened the pill bottle. My mind was blank, and my heart was shut off. All I wanted to do was go to sleep and not wake up.

I'm not sure when or why I woke up, but when I did, I found myself over the toilet bowl vomiting. I quickly realized that my plan had not worked and slowly I began coming back to reality like a veil being lifted from my face. Not wanting to end up with liver damage, I took a cab to the hospital. I told them I had accidentally taken too many pills, however blood tests showed that I had *no* drugs in my body whatsoever, so they didn't believe me. I was filled with shame over what I had done and at the same time I had trouble believing it had actually happened. Then, after I insisted to the social worker that it really was an accident, they sent me home. Dazed, I walked ten kilometers back home and went to bed. I was in shock that no drugs had showed up in my system, and wondered how that was possible. For all intense purposes, with the type of narcotics I took, and how many of them I had taken, it made no sense that I was still alive with no side effects whatsoever. It would be many years before I would realize that God had a different plan for my life.

The next morning, void of emotion, I went to work like nothing had happened. No one knew a thing. My deep depression had ended and all thoughts about wanting to end my life had vanished. People in my life seemed to think that I really had my act together, and wondered why I was always so positive and happy.

I had become quite a good actress, but I was not good enough to convince myself.

One good thing came of that incident. I realized that I needed help, and I found a psychologist, Dr. Moniker. He was new to the field of psychoanalysis, but very kind; in fact, I believe I was his first real psychoanalysis case. At first, I had trouble taking off my mask with him because I didn't want him thinking I was crazy and I didn't want to feel judged. I also felt very ashamed about all of my suicide attempts. Because even though I had done it and surly I had emotional issues that had to be dealt with, it didn't really feel like it had been *me* wanting to end my life. Eventually Dr. Moniker was able to break down my walls. He seemed like he really wanted to help me and see things through so, when I couldn't afford to pay for treatment, he offered to see me for free and in return he would write about me in one of his books. He was the only person I felt comfortable enough with to be honest about how I was feeling. While I played the victim role quite well, I just wanted to love and be loved, and had found that the people in my life did not seem capable of that.

When I started seeing Dr. Moniker I was able to delve into my childhood, and to explore how I was self-sabotaging my emotional life in order to sustain my belief that I did not deserve anything good out of life. I learned that I believed what my parents had told me; that I was stupid and worthless. Although they likely did not really mean those things, my subconscious wanted to fulfill what I had heard them say, and in doing so I was somehow honoring them.

This concept was hard to digest, and left me wondering how I could ever start to believe in myself, or go so far as to even like myself? Apparently, I subconsciously chose men who would hurt me, or who were emotionally unavailable, despite consciously wanting more. This was so that I could stay true to my parents, who also had been emotionally unavailable. But why would I want to sabotage myself like that? Was I that messed up? I grappled with this concept and sort of accepted it on a surface level, but it really didn't sink in on a deeper level. Evidently, a lot more heartbreak would be required.

I would see Dr. Moniker on and off for over 10 years. Sometimes life got busy, or sometimes I needed time to process things on my own. I felt he was like a friend of sorts, who was always there to lead me straight back into reality and out of my fantasy land, and he accepted me without judgment. I could tell him the ugly thoughts that ran through me, and he never once looked down his nose at me. He tried to get me to believe I was worthy of so much more, but it was a hard sell. Then, after a two-year break from therapy, I tried to go back and see him again but found out that he'd got cancer and died rather quickly.

He was the only person who ever really knew me, and I was very sad to hear of his death. I often wonder what he would have written about me in his book that he never got to finish.

Juan 2.0

If I seem detached and matter-of-fact in my writing, it's because that is how I managed my life—at least on the exterior—at that time. I walked through much of my life on autopilot, operating only on a surface level. I was expert at quickly dismissing any awareness of the struggles that plagued me beneath the surface.

How could I want to self-sabotage, as Dr. Moniker said, even if it was on an unconscious level? Was there some kind of 'self-destruct' button in my brain that I was secretly playing with? Rather than delving into the mess inside me, it was easier to just stay busy and avoid such confusing thoughts. I tried to convince myself that I was strong, and that I was a kind, loving regular gal. I went out with friends, got back together with Juan, and did a lot of salsa dancing. I got a second job teaching others to dance, and I would also perform and compete.

Dancing kept me busy and shut out the voices in my head. When I danced, the world went quiet and the voice that relished in telling me how worthless I was became silent. Instead, it was just me and the music, which brought me to life. I could be anyone I wanted to be when I danced.

Salsa dancing was magic to me, despite that I sustained a couple of minor concussions. I dreamt of making it a full-time career. One night I was dancing with Juan and somehow my nose met his elbow during a fast turn. My nose not only broke, but it shifted out of place. I ran into the bathroom and set the bone back into place before the swelling got too bad, but I ended up needing surgery to fix it.

Ultimately, I can't remember why I ever got back together with Juan—maybe because I thought we could still salvage our 'marriage'. Then I became pregnant. When I told him, he cried and begged me to have an abortion—the first and last time I would see him cry. I adamantly refused. My conscience just wouldn't let me do what he wanted me to do. We broke up and I told him that I would raise the baby on my own. I was very sad about the situation, but at the same time something inside me was growing, and now I felt like I had a purpose in life. I knew I could be a good mother, and I welcomed the idea that when the baby was born, I would have someone I could love who wouldn't run away. It hurt so much to break up because I'd hoped this would unite us.

Around that time my parents announced that they were getting a divorce. It was a shock, but it was also kind of a relief. Neither of them were happy, and it made me nauseous to see how badly my mother treated my father. She would walk around with this scowl on her face and on many occasions I heard her muttering under her breath how stupid he was. By this time, my father had become very gentle and passive, and so he just took whatever my mother doled out and never said a thing. Although she never admitted it, I believe my mother had an affair, because I occasionally caught her chatting online with a man. She said they were just friends, but when she went away on a 'business trip', I knew she was lying. She had never been on a business trip before, and her job did not require that type of travel. Years later my suspicions were confirmed when she let something slip. But who was I to judge?

In the meantime, I felt sorry for my dad. Sure, he wasn't the greatest husband. He lived in his own bubble of religion, work, music, and literature. Their conversations were nothing but superficial, and my mom did virtually all of the housework. Perhaps she felt unappreciated. All I can say is that no one knows what really goes on in a relationship except for the two people in the relationship, and even then, each will have their own biased view.

Over the years each of my parents have each divulged to me various details of their married life, and each has their own version. Both have, at different times, demonstrated traits of martyrdom and victim syndrome. At the time they were separating, however, my dad most definitely was the victim, and he needed my support most. He was absolutely devastated, while my mother seemed to be very happy. Dad never imagined that my mother would leave him, and he absolutely did not know how to cope. Ultimately, I became the shoulder he cried on. It was a strange feeling for me, because I was providing the support to him that I never received as a child because 'feelings' were not something we ever discussed in our home. It did make us closer. It felt good to be needed.

In the midst of this chaos and uncertainty, I knew it was time to tell my parents about the baby. I was scared they would once again disown me as they had in the past, but there was no choice. My relationship with them had been improving, and I think when I asked to speak to them they both thought I had called them together to try to help them patch things up between them.

We sat in the living room, my mother with her arms crossed and a slight scowl on her face, my father passive and numb, just waiting to hear what I had to say. I was nervous, but excited at the same time. What a bomb to drop. "Mom, Dad... I'm pregnant. And oh, by the way, I got married a year ago but we just broke up."

The silence in the room became even more uncomfortable. There were coughs and splutters as they tried to figure out what to say. Nick, my brother, piped up and said, "Why don't you just get an abortion?"

My dad lost it. He got up and yelled at Nick. "That is an abomination to God! That is murdering an innocent life! You should be supporting your sister because she is being brave and having this baby on her own."

I almost fell off my chair. My father... *supporting* me? This was going better than I could ever have hoped. My mother chimed in and said that I would not be alone, and that they would help me in whatever way they could. I suppose she was relieved I wasn't playing 'marriage counselor' with them. It was quite surprising to me to have both of their support. I felt like a large weight had been taken off my chest, and so I left them to talk. I was going to start a new chapter in my life.

Juan called me a month later and told me that he would 'try' to be a father and a husband. I was hesitant, but agreed to take him back. A few months later, we moved into an apartment together. It was in a great location and had a great view. Up until then, I had never told Juan that I loved him, for fear that it would scare him off; however, on our first night in our new place, I could not hold my feelings for him back anymore, and so I mustered up all the courage I had and, with his baby growing inside me, said, "I love you."

He gently took my sweaty palms into his hands and looked into my eyes as I held my breath in anticipation. Then, speaking softly and sweetly, he told me that although I was nice, sweet and that he liked me, he would never be able to love me because he didn't think he was capable of loving anyone. He told me he had never wanted a family, but that he would do his best to be a good husband and father and that maybe in time he would learn to love me.

I sat in stunned silence, trying to hold back tears, smiling at him like this was all great—but inside my heart broke into pieces. Something in me died that night when I agreed to those terms, and I was so angry with myself. I told him I understood, and that I was really tired and needed to sleep and I went to bed. I could not exactly fault him for not pledging his undying love; he'd told me when he met me that he never wanted to settle down, but I had pushed anyway, thinking I could make him magically fall in love with me and abandon his desire of eternal bachelorhood. I had convinced myself that if I had fit myself into a mold I thought he wanted, he would love me—but I had failed.

As time went on, I pushed these feelings aside, but one part of me hung on to the hope that he could love me one day, another part of me kept telling me that this was the best I could do because I didn't deserve love, and yet *another* part of me reasoned that my baby needed its father ... and I did not want to do it alone. Meanwhile, Juan remained polite but detached. He was rarely home and when he was, he would come in late and then go straight to bed. As for me, I still had two jobs, a full-time job at an insurance company and part-time job teaching dance. When I wasn't working, I busied myself decorating our apartment in preparation for our baby and reading books on how to be a mother.

My beautiful baby girl came into the world on a cold November day after 24 hours of labor. I had been out dancing the night before at a ballroom nightclub with my dance students, and I imagine this had something to do with the fact that she was born three weeks before her due date.

I want to say that I looked at her and fell in love in an instant, but instead I felt kind of numb ... and then I felt guilty. I now held this wonderful life in my arms, and wanted to give her everything, but my 'husband' didn't love me. He was just playing family because he believed it was the right thing to do. As people came to visit, I said and did all the things a new mother is supposed to do. I showed off my beautiful baby with pride, but sadness crept into my heart. How could I be a mother? This angel deserved better than the parents she got stuck with. Naturally, I never told anyone how I felt. Thank goodness the feeling passed within a couple of weeks. Looking back, I think that perhaps it was, at least in part, postpartum depression.

Soon I was spending long days alone with my little girl. I fell in love with her. She needed me and I liked feeling needed.

It felt good to have a purpose and it was such a joy to be around her. She was such an easy baby to take care of. I became 'mother extraordinaire'. My whole world revolved around her and I stopped caring that my husband was hardly ever home. We went to parks and playgroups, went on long walks, and spent lots of time giggling on the living room floor with toys, singing, and reading. None of my friends had children so it was pretty lonely, but in a way, I was reinventing my own childhood by enjoying hers so much. It made me happy to do silly things to make her laugh.

Juan was less involved with our daughter, and he pursued his own interests. In retrospect, it was almost inevitable that eventually I found a pair of women's underwear that did not belong to me in our laundry. Shaking with fear as I waited for him to come home that night, I confronted him and he told me they must have been left in the apartment machine by the person who'd used it before us. He told me that he would never cheat, and asked me how I could possibly think this of him. He was so convincing that I felt guilty for accusing him … and yet, deep inside I knew he was cheating. A woman knows such things, and whether we admit it to ourselves or not, it doesn't make it less true. However, I decided to let it go because I was scared of being a single mother, of having a broken family, of being alone and of feeling like a failure.

Juan continued to work long hours, but was getting depressed by his job. An opportunity came up for him to work in Spain doing sales. The job didn't sound too great, but the thought of starting over and having a new life was exciting, so I agreed to go there with him to live. He went first to Portugal for two months training before moving on to Spain to find a place for us to live. During that time I sold all of our apartment furniture and moved in with my dad.

Juan came back two months later, after deciding that the job was not what he thought it would be. So, with no place to stay and no furniture, we decided to stay with my dad while we saved up money. It was only supposed to be for one year, but we ended up staying for six. I have to say that despite their earlier failings, my parents were absolutely wonderful and so supportive. My dad was overjoyed to have his granddaughter close by, and my brother Nick thought she was the most wonderful little girl in the world. He always spoiled her with gifts whenever he came over.

Going back to work after maternity leave was so incredibly hard for me. I reduced my hours so I could be with my daughter. I couldn't bear the thought of someone else raising her. She was such a joy to be around. Her exotic Latina looks, combined with her radiant smile and sunny disposition, just tore at my heartstrings.

By the time my daughter turned two, Juan still hadn't proclaimed his love for me. I still felt so alone, yet I was growing stronger. I mustered up the courage to tell him that if he didn't love me, our relationship was over. I didn't want to remain married anymore to someone who didn't love me. This was not an example of marriage that I wanted to model for my daughter. Besides, my self-esteem had been getting a boost lately. Men had started noticing me and flirting with me again when I went out, and it felt good to be desired and noticed. I told Juan that he had one month to decide what he wanted to do. If he was sure that he did not love me, then he could leave.

Eventually, Juan mustered a lackluster, "I love you." It was hard for him to do it. I'm not sure whether it was true or not, but I accepted it and hoped things would get better, which they did for a time. Prior to this, Juan had been unemployed for a while, and while trying to figure out what he wanted to do, he'd got into online trading. When that turned out not to be as fruitful as he'd hoped, he got a job as a welder. That was more lucrative, and it was nice to be able to pay off some of debts. Along with becoming a better earner, he also became a more attentive father. We settled into a routine which, while it didn't provide much emotional connection, generated some fun along the way.

In an attempt to rekindle some romance between us, Juan suggested we try watching pornography. He told me that his fantasy was to watch me with another woman. Deep down, it felt wrong to me, but I wanted to feel desired by him again and I was willing to try to make my husband happy. We started going to 'swing clubs', and while we did not do any 'swinging', I did dance provocatively with a very attractive woman and we kissed in front of everyone. Our love life improved, as Juan returned home aroused after those nights at the club. Still, it felt empty to me. All he could talk about was seeing me with another woman, and it felt that it was not *me* he really desired. This was confusing, because our love life had been utterly amazing throughout our relationship, right up until the time I became pregnant.

My therapist told me that some men are no longer attracted to their wives after they become mothers, or after watching them give birth. I tried to rationalize this. In my role as a paramedic, I had delivered many babies and I understood that what happens to a woman's body during delivery is not what one would describe as sexy. I wondered if the swinger's club was what Juan needed in order to see me as a woman again, and not just as a mother, and so I decided to stick it out as a way to entice him and strengthen our intimacy. But then, he wanted more. Juan said he wanted to go to a different kind of club where people could watch us during our lovemaking, a place where he could watch me with another woman. Still wanting to please him, I agreed.

The lifestyle of couples sharing intimacy with other people while still staying together in committed relationships was a whole new world to me. Between the adrenaline rush that came from having new, potentially dangerous experiences and the reaction of my hormones to the situation, it was exciting. Both men and women in the club desired me because I had a great figure and I guess you could say I was pretty. It lifted my fragile ego to hear how hot and sexy I was from strangers. I drowned out my conscience, thinking to myself, *maybe Juan will notice me and find me desirable now …*

I assumed that people who went to such places were sex-crazed weirdos, but I couldn't have been more wrong. It was surprising for me to learn that many of the people who went there had children, respectable jobs, and were genuinely nice, decent people. Most said they had very good marriages that were enhanced because they allowed themselves to indulge in this kind of 'play' together. One couple said they had been on the brink of divorce until they started coming to the club, and that swinging had opened up communication for them and ultimately strengthened their marriage. I pondered whether this could happen to Juan and me. Maybe I could do this; maybe I could just let my inhibitions go and adopt this kind of life—after all, it was just my body. However, I just could not ignore the lead weight in my stomach and the fact that after leaving the club I felt used, dirty, empty, and cheap.

When I confessed these feelings to Juan, he admitted that although he'd had momentary pangs of guilt about the experience, he'd really liked it. Something was stirring inside of him, it seemed, and out of the blue he suggested that we have another child. I was shocked, but hopeful that this would save our marriage, so I said 'yes', and I became pregnant again very quickly. However, the pregnancy did nothing for our marriage; instead, things started to deteriorate. Prior to the pregnancy, things had finally been moving in the right direction with us, but when I got pregnant, I told him I would not be going to those clubs any longer. Our relationship was quickly reduced to superficial conversations and pleasantries, with no intimacy of any type.

We began to have a series of meaningless arguments that never resolved, because Juan would abruptly walk away from me and refuse to speak to me for days. Then, just as abruptly, he would behave like it had never happened and that everything was fine. However, the silent treatments and unresolved issues began slowly eating away at me. The words 'I love you' that I had longed to hear from him became just that—words. There was no feeling behind them. I regressed to feeling incredibly empty.

We barely spoke. There was practically no affection between us, although he never outwardly treated me badly, and our family and friends saw us as a happy couple. The one thing we did have in common was to keep up appearances of happiness to the outside world. I think the moment I knew it was over between Juan and I was the day I gave birth to our youngest daughter. Right after she arrived, Juan went straight to a chair in the corner of the room, covered himself in a blanket and went to sleep. After hours of intense labor and delivery, not a single acknowledgement was uttered—not so much as a kiss, or a 'way to go, honey' were provided to me.

I sat nursing my newborn in tears, glad to have another beautiful baby girl, but in despair for my marriage. I was both overjoyed at being a parent again and deeply lonely as I realized that Juan could not, and would not, love me as I wanted to be loved. He wanted to be a man of honor, and that was why he had stayed with me and our child, but his heart was not in it. I looked at my new baby daughter and felt so much love for her, but I also felt anger and resentment—not only toward Juan, but toward myself for continuing to live in a dream world. It would take me a couple of years to understand that he cared for me the only way he knew how, and that he just was not meant to be in a marriage.

A couple of months after my second daughter was born, I was presented with the opportunity of a lifetime. I had dreamed of dancing in the Brazilian carnival ever since I'd been a little girl and had found a picture of a Brazilian woman, in full dance costume, in a book … and now I had been offered an audition! I had never danced a Brazilian carnival samba before but with my dance background, combined with intense training, I was in top form in a few months. The dance school was very surprised that a non-Brazilian could dance samba so well, and I was delighted when they accepted me! They said they were excited to have a Canadian dancer.

I couldn't believe my luck. Juan and I packed up the kids and went to Brazil so I could train with the school, even though I had some hip pain before we left. There was no way I was going to let that stop me, so I found a sports medicine doctor who agreed to inject steroids into the muscle, which seemed to help.

When I'd first talked about this opportunity with Juan, he'd been very supportive of my venture, even helping make travel and accommodation arrangements, as it afforded him the opportunity to spend time with his Brazilian family. However, I was quite taken aback at how his demeanor changed when he saw my costume—a barely-there bikini thong, itty bitty bra, and big, full headdress. Because he'd grown up in Brazil and was used to such costumes, I'd assumed he would be okay with my participation in the carnival; instead, he was jealous! I had never seen him jealous before. Did this mean he loved me?

His reaction was to decide that he wanted to take part in the carnival too. He could not be a dancer, but he could be part of the parade. This made me angry because it felt like he was stealing my moment, and that he didn't want me to be happy. It was unsettling that, after paying me no attention in our domestic life, he suddenly didn't want other men looking at me. He became a real watchdog. He came to all my rehearsals and began following me around like he was marking his territory. Up until then, he'd never cared what I wore or where I went. What had changed, and why now?

We fought and didn't talk much, which took some of the wind out of my sails, but I refused to give up this dream of mine. I just wanted to dance, and though Juan's presence irked me, when I danced it felt like magic!

The samba school had a very large arena to practice in, but even its vast size could not hold all the participants, who were decked out in wildly lavish, exquisitely detailed costumes. The sound of about 50 drummers, which in Brazil is called a 'batteria'—is all encompassing, especially when it is in an indoor arena. The drums pounding becomes the very heartbeat in your chest. When it is then mixed with the entire school singing, it is absolutely thrilling. We dancers had to sing as well as dance, and we were right in front of the batteria. It was exhilarating, and every day after practice, though my legs throbbed in pain, I was filled with adrenaline charged joy.

The day of the parade came. I was nervous because, as a pale Northerner, I stood out like a sore thumb ... which meant many eyes would be on me once we hit the dance floor. Our school went on at 4:00 a.m., and to this day, dancing for that one hour—in three-inch platform heels, in front of millions of people, on live TV—still stands out as the most exhilarating and physically exhausting experience of my life! I was not the best dancer by far, but I held my own. Unfortunately, the steroid injection I had before I went to Brazil actually made my hip worse, and it hurt like heck the whole time I danced—but it was worth it.

At the time, it was not common to have foreigners as Carnival dancers, though it is more common now, but at the time, I was a novelty and so some people wanted to have me on the news, because it was a big deal for a Canadian to be dancing Brazilian Carnival Samba. I refused. I had fulfilled one of my dreams, and that was enough. I didn't want the spotlight or attention.

When we returned to Canada, things went back to the way they had been before. Eventually I came to understand that Juan, much like myself, had come from a long line of brokenness. Appearances meant everything to him, which is likely the reason why he didn't want a divorce, even though he didn't really want me. We lived unhappily this way for almost two years, barely touching and barely speaking. During this time, I tried to convince him to go to counseling, but he refused. I also tried to get him to go back to salsa dancing with me, but he didn't want to. So I started going out by myself once a week, and that empty void in my heart began to fill a little when I met Dan.

Dan wanted to go into professional dancing, and he wanted me as his dance partner. We trained hard and I envisioned myself as a professional dancer. I even fantasized about being with Dan because I knew he was attracted to me. However, that dream of professional dancing quickly became shattered when I started having severe hip pain and could not move my leg. I began the rounds of doctors, and three top specialists all gave me different answers as to why I could not externally rotate my left leg; if I tried, the pain was excruciating. They said my symptoms and tests did not fit normal patterns of any known problems, and tests and X-rays came back showing only very mild arthritis. However, I persisted in getting professional opinions, because I knew deep inside that something was very wrong.

Finally, I found Dr. Number Four, who said my hip was growing bone in places where it shouldn't be, and the two bones were trying to fuse themselves together. The problem, he said, could only be corrected with arthroscopic hip surgery, in which they shave off the bony overgrowth, and as this was a relatively new procedure, there was only one surgeon in the city who could perform the surgery. The bad news was that the wait time for this surgery was 18 months.

This was unacceptable to me. I already had pain in my heart from my soulless marriage, and I would not tolerate the pain in my hip any longer. Besides, I was contemplating leaving my husband, and I knew I could not be an effective single parent if I was unable to move my leg.

I wanted the problem to go away quickly, so I did some research ... and two weeks later I was out on the opposite end of the country having the surgery, with my mother by my side to help. She had graciously offer to accompany me because it would have been impossible for me to go alone and Juan needed to stay home with the children. I tried so hard to not show any pain to my mom so that she would not worry so instead I filled myself with narcotics. Unfortunately, after the surgery, the doctors told me that the damage to my hip was severe. The labrum (cartilage) was shredded and couldn't be repaired. They had shaved off the parts of the bones that had tried to fuse together, they told me, but the arthritis was very bad. They said I was eventually going to need a hip replacement, though I was too young for it yet, and advised me to try to delay that procedure as long as possible.

I was bewildered. All of my scans and tests had come back showing a normal hip, and yet this doctor was telling me that mine was one of the worst he had seen in someone my age. At the same time, it was oddly comforting to know this, because other doctors had told me there was nothing wrong. There was some satisfaction in knowing that my instincts had been right. I was discouraged, but at least the pain was more tolerable.

I went back home to complete my recovery, and had no help whatsoever from my roommate husband who was busy trying to 'get rich quick' through online trading schemes. I immersed myself in treatment and medication, and while I regained more use of my leg, there was still pain.

I was still on crutches when Juan brought Brian home one day. Brian was my daughter's soccer coach, and Juan hoped that Brian and his wife could be our new friends. Brian and I had an instant connection. For the first time in many years, someone talked to me and was interested in what I had to say. Brian was also very spiritual, in a new age kind of way, which I found attractive. Finding a deeper meaning in my life was a hidden yearning that had been brewing inside of me for years, and so when Brian opened that door for me, I was like a moth to a flame. Coincidentally, Brian was going through the same situation with his wife that I was going through with Juan, and he was searching, as I was, for a deeper connection. We became friends, and soon Brian and I were getting together with for playdates with our daughters while our respective spouses worked. By now I knew I had to leave Juan. He didn't really love me and I had given up trying to win him over. Brian was my charming prince!

The flirtation with Brian was electric, and I could hardly wait to be with him. I was surprised at how easily Juan agreed when I asked him for a divorce. However, he needed time to save up money to move out, so we lived together for nine more months, which was a very tense time for the both of us. Finally, when it came time for him to move out, reality hit him, and he panicked, although to this day I think it was less about the fear of losing me, and more about the fear of becoming a single father. He tried to negotiate by offering me oral sex once a week, as well as promising that we would have sex together more often. *Really? Is that what he thought it would take??* Then he claimed he really *did* love me but didn't know how to show it, and even offered to go to counseling. But after seven years of trying so hard to make things work, there was nothing left inside me anymore for him. I had wished for so long that he would agree to counseling, and I felt very sad for him—but for me, it was now too late. I was already in love with Brian. Brian was an artist and a musician, and we could talk for hours, while Juan and I had never really been able to talk, not about anything of substance at least.

I told Juan 'no'. It was over. In my heart, I was certain that Brian was going to be my new happily ever after.

Brian

'Happily ever after' turned out to be more like 'nightmare ever after'. When all was said and done, it turned out Brian was just using me to get out of his marriage, and he thought I could be his next sugar mama. Sadly, it took me *way* too long to figure this out.

Brian had been a male model a few years prior to us meeting. Although he was very slim and not athletic at all, there was something so sexy about him. Maybe it was that he oozed the self-confidence that I was so lacking in. With his bald head, and smoldering blue eyes, he just had this sexy lustful look to him. We jumped right in, head over heels, in lust with each other.

Alarm bells should have gone off the moment I saw the amount of 'stuff' Brian had. He came with so much physical baggage that I cannot even describe it. Hoarders had *nothing* on this guy! A large storage room stacked to the ceiling would not be enough to hold just the boxes of old papers and junk that he'd accumulated and couldn't deal with. Unfortunately for me, I didn't clue into the fact that if someone has THAT much physical baggage, they are likely to be carrying an equal amount of emotional baggage. What can I say? Love, or at least infatuation, is blind!

My daughters had a hard time adjusting to the separation at first, and so I insisted on equal shared custody. Though it tore my heart not to be with my girls every day, I knew they needed their father as much as they needed me, and it was the right thing to do. I swore to myself I would not let my personal feelings towards Juan affect the relationship they had with their father. So many divorces get ugly, and children end up suffering the most. I wasn't going to let that happen.

I had my doubts about whether I had done the right thing in divorcing Juan, but I truly felt that my girls needed to witness a marriage filled with love—and that was not what Juan and I had. I was still living at my dad's house when Juan moved out and was planning on living with my dad for one more year, but only three weeks into my separation my dad found out I was dating Brian and told me that he would not tolerate me treating 'his' son that way and that I had to leave his house.

I was hurt—wasn't I his daughter? And here he was, once again, siding with someone else? The feeling of being betrayed and abandoned by my parents once came back to haunt me. I thought my dad had changed, and that our relationship had improved over the past seven years while we'd lived under the same roof. I can only suppose that my separation from Juan reminded of his own divorce and triggered an emotional response, that of the poor helpless man whose wife left. But this time, his rejection of me did not hurt nearly as much as being disowned all those years ago had. I had my daughters, and I was going to start a new life.

A few months later, I bought a house one block away from my dad's house because I wanted my girls to be in a familiar environment close to their neighborhood friends and school. I felt excited to start over. I had always been extremely savvy with my finances, and the house was a great price because it was a true fixer upper. Brian and I immediately decided that we had to live together. In retrospect, I am pretty sure it was him convincing me that we had to be together all the time and me, being in the lost state that I was, just went along with it. Brian moved into the basement with his daughter, who had halftime custody of in a similar arrangement to the one I'd made with Juan. We were together as a couple, but we agreed to keep our relationship secret from the kids for at least one year in order to give them a chance to adjust.

Everyone seemed excited about the move, and once we were in the new house, I began to work on it. I painted everything mostly on my own, which was cathartic in a way. Meanwhile, it felt good to be in love. Brian told me I was his soul mate, which made me weak in the knees. I was convinced he was mine. I felt so in tune with him that it was like we could read each other's thoughts, and I was so attracted to this man that it blurred everything else. For example, I was unfazed by the fact that he was unemployed, because I wanted to believe he would someday be a rock star and earn lots of money.

Brian was the first musician I had ever been with, so to me he was incredible, though I would come to understand in time that he wasn't really that good. He didn't work because he'd suffered a concussion in a car accident not long before we met. He said it was his intent to go back to work once he got better, but he never did—and not because of his supposed concussion, but because he was lazy.

At first, before I discovered these things, I was devoted to being the most faithful, wonderful, perfect girlfriend. I supported him, paid his bills, and became his little servant. He claimed to be depressed and convinced me that catering to him was what I would do as someone who loved him. And I obliged.

I also spent a lot of time with the children. I made the basement into a big playroom and fairly soon my house became the place where all the neighborhood kids wanted to be, and it filled me with joy. We had dance parties, played games, made plays, and went to parks. Once, my eldest daughter asked me why I spent so much time doing things with them when her friends' mothers did not. I told her that I loved being with them, and that I didn't have children so *other* people could raise them, but so that *I* could. To this day, I cherish those years so much.

While Juan and I divorced somewhat amicably, Brian wound up in the middle of a nasty divorce and custody battle. He asked me to help him, and so I did. It felt good to be needed; Juan had never reached out to me in such a vulnerable way.

Help mostly took the form of filling out paperwork and going to court hearings with him. Brian had me convinced that his ex-wife was pure evil, which was supported by the fact that his daughter didn't want to be with her mother. Of course, not only did his daughter and my eldest get along very well, but our home was fun, which may have swayed the girl.

Brian had a very relaxed parenting style. He believed that kids needed space to discover their authentic selves, and that they would not flourish if they had too many rules. This view appealed to me because I had grown up with nothing *but* rules and control, and I did not want to repeat the pattern with my own children. Ultimately, for a while it felt like we were really a team and that we were helping each other; I was helping with his custody and insurance stuff, and he with helping me to open up more and share my feelings, which I had been used to bottling up. It felt good to learn to let myself be vulnerable again.

But it didn't last. Things seemed to be going along well, but suddenly Brian began to be somewhat distant. I also noted he was on his computer a fair bit, and he'd started going out more often on his own. We were connecting less and less. Had I done something wrong?

It was around a year into the relationship that I caught Brian cheating. I was suspicious of a relationship he had with a woman he referred to as a 'friend', and when I confronted her she admitted an affair—although she had been under the impression that he was single.

I approached Brian and told him I knew what was going on, but he managed to twist the situation around and make it seem like it was *my* fault. He said I was not really opening myself up enough to him, and that he needed more. He also claimed he was so depressed he didn't know what he was doing. Then he said I was really special, but that I was, "a diamond covered in shit," and that my 'holding back' made him feel like I didn't really love him. He was referring to the fact that I refused to add his name to my bank account, or put his name on the title of the house. Some little voice inside me had told me not to share my finances with him, though Brian insisted we could never really share a life together and be true partners if I wouldn't share everything with him. I felt guilty when he cried and told me he just wanted us to really belong to each other and he did not really want anyone else.

It was hard to resist Brian. He was also good with kids, and was a children's soccer coach, which made him doubly attractive to me. As I looked into his weepy bedroom eyes, I told him I would think about it. Looking back, perhaps I was just gullible and naive—but he was such a convincing liar! And truth be told, he had the power to get to me because I had started to believe his stories about how flawed I was, and my inner voice was telling me that if I had been more vulnerable to him, he would not have needed to cheat. I also kept thinking about the incredible connection we'd initially had, and though it had only lasted a few months, I wanted that closeness back.

As the darkness closed in, I was sure I would never find anything close to that 'in love with my soul mate' feeling I'd had with Brian, let alone find a man who *really* loved me. One night, the darkness returned and depression over this situation hit me out of nowhere like a Mack truck. I became angry at Brian, and felt so betrayed—but even more, I felt like my life was just one huge failure, and I had let everyone down.

Feelings of worthlessness consumed me, and I began to drown in self-loathing. All I'd wanted was a loving relationship that would show my kids what a good, solid partnership looked like—but I couldn't even do that right. My mind was spinning with thought about how much of a failure as a mother I was. I felt like no one in my life truly saw me, or cared about me. Intrusive thoughts that I would be better off dead consumed me, and told me that no one would miss me anyway. *The kids have their father, and they'll eventually be fine without me,* I told myself. *I have to leave this pathetic life.*

The plunge into that rabbit hole happened in only one hour. Brian was asleep, my kids were with their dad for a few days and I did not want to feel the pain in my heart anymore. I went into that old familiar trance-like robotic state, and soon found myself naked in the bathtub with a razor blade. As with my previous suicide attempt, I left no note. I was consumed only with a desire to get it over with quickly, and end my life. I drew the sharp blade over the vein in my wrist, barely even feeling the pain. I stared transfixed at the blood gushing out, almost like a fountain. It felt like I was watching a movie.

The water turned red very quickly, but I hardly noticed it. The world just went so still and quiet. I felt relief as I my life slowly drained out of me. I don't remember how long I stayed that way, but suddenly something snapped in me and brought me back to reality. I didn't want to die! What if my kids found me like this? It would traumatize and scar them so deeply. What if I wasn't as bad as I though? What if those voices whispering in my ear how worthless I was, were wrong?

I quickly applied pressure to the wound, but I was weak after losing so much blood, and I could not stand up. I tried shouting out to Brian, but he did not hear me and so I began to panic. *What if I can't get up? What if I can't stop the bleeding?*

I removed my hand from the wound and the blood came flowing back out. I looked down at my body and saw I was covered in thick, red blood. I wanted to throw up. I felt confused, disoriented and bewildered at what I had done. I screamed as loud as my weak voice would go, and then Brian walked into the room. All he could say was, "Holy shit!" It must have been quite a shock for him to see because it looked like a scene out of a gruesome murder, with blood sprayed all over the walls.

I asked him to help me out of the tub and he did, and then I collapsed on the floor, still holding on to my wrist for dear life. He told me he was going to call 911, but I begged him not to. The fog in my brain had cleared and I did not want to end up in a psych ward, or have my family find out what I had done. It would be too humiliating. This wasn't really who I was! There was no way I wanted to be labeled as crazy. "No," I told him, "I can do this. I have the training."

I would not find out until our relationship had truly ended that while I was lying on the ground, Brian used his cell phone to snap pictures of me, which he would later use to try to blackmail me (though it never worked). You have to be extremely cold-hearted to take pictures in a moment like that.

Brian helped me to my bed. I lay in his arms and sobbed at what I had done, and I made him promise not to tell anyone. For two days he cared for me, cooked for me and told me how much he loved me. We talked and laughed like we'd done when we'd first met. He even promised to get help with finding a job. I buried my feelings of anger, shame, guilt, and self-loathing, and I told myself I had my soul mate back.

My wound healed quickly, and by the third day, I was back to physical health. I felt like we'd turned a page, and I returned to loving and doting on him like nothing had ever happened. All the while, unbeknownst to me, he returned to cheating and lying about it. With so many failed relationships in my past, I was determined to make this one work. All I wanted was my 'happily ever after'. Eventually the cheating got to be too much for me. I tried to talk to him about my feelings but he refused to discuss it, saying that we had to move forward. He also told me I would never be able to find someone else and—because of the little voice in my head telling me not to expect better, because I wasn't good enough, or pretty enough—I believed him.

Brian used to go away for days at a time to 'clear his head'. The last straw for me in our relationship came on a weekend when he decided to 'clear his head' instead of attending to his responsibilities. I had gone away up north for the weekend with some friends, and he was supposed to meet us there ... but he never showed up. I came home two days later to find that he'd probably vacated the house the minute I did—and he'd left his dog alone in my house the whole time. The poor dog soiled himself everywhere, and there were piles of dog poop all over my house. I was livid.

I tried to hunt him down by phone, but he was unreachable. I drove the dog over to his dad's house, all the while entertaining fleeting thoughts of letting it loose in a park somewhere—but of course, it was not the dog's fault.

This was the last straw. I had finally come to my senses, and I was done with Brian. I worked tirelessly for two days straight to bring all his boxes out of my basement and into my carport. The carport was overflowing, so I put the rest in the yard and told him to come to get them or they'd go into the garbage. He never came. He texted that he was sorry, that he was in a bad emotional state and that he would be back soon. He said his cell phone had died, and that he'd gotten lost.

There was no way I was going to believe that, and there was no way that I was going to let him come back into my house, so I changed the locks, paid one month's worth of storage fees, and moved all of his things into a storage unit. Moving his junk was no easy feat due to the sheer volume of it all, and so I was lucky to have some dear friends to help me.

I tried to cover the hurt and sadness that plagued my heart, and keeping busy helped me. I could not help but notice that somehow the house felt so much lighter with Brian gone. I did not miss him, but I ached over the loss of what I thought, or hoped, our relationship could have been. As I healed, slowly my heart let go of the fantasy that there is such a thing as a soul mate, but the idea was crushing and terrifying, and it left a giant hole in my chest, akin to a mother giving up her child.

I wondered, *what is the purpose of life without a soul mate? Could all those romance movies and books be wrong?* I'd never wanted a fancy house or clothes, or anything that money could buy. I'd always just wanted to find a soul mate to complete me, my perfect other half. Realizing that such a one did not exist, and the connectedness I craved would never happen, I was suddenly at a loss as to what to do with myself. I felt like I was in a dark room searching for a light switch. I began to think about God, about the God of my childhood, and the God of the Christian woman who'd come to me to tell me Juan was cheating on me. I never doubted he was real, but now I wondered, *where is God in all of this? Does He even care about my troubles? Did He see this wretched lonely pain deep within my soul?* I prayed, but I heard no answer.

A neighbor, whose daughter was friends with my daughters, saw my state and began inviting me over to family dinners, and checking in on me regularly. On the surface, I tried to be the same friendly, light-hearted person people knew me as, but she knew some of the things that had happened and saw the hopelessness in my eyes. Her support and compassion, along with that of a few other friends, got me thinking that perhaps there was hope for me after all. Perhaps I *didn't* need another half to make me whole. Maybe I was whole on my own.

To this day, I don't think my neighbor and friends know that it was their love and kindness that saved me and give me hope to carry on. Their unselfish love dulled the nasty voices inside my head that kept telling me that I was worthless. Their support gave me the strength to trudge on, and to feel less overwhelmed by the idea of being finally and truly on my own.

Brian had left behind seven really expensive guitars. A girlfriend of mine kept saying I should sell them to recover all the money he had taken from me, but something in me just couldn't do it. I was determined not to sink to his level, and to instead act with love—not toward him specifically, but toward a fellow lost soul. I didn't want to be a person consumed by thoughts of revenge; I did not have much compassion left inside me, but I could choose to be fair.

On the night Brian came to get his stuff, I holed up at a neighbor's house so that I would not have to see him with his new girlfriend. I left all his things intact, as I felt I should. This chapter of my life with Brian in it was closed for good. A sense of peace trickled over me.

Pat

I decided to take a few months away from dating to get my feet on the ground. It seemed like a healthy thing to do. I thought, *there has to be something more to life than just falling in and out of love and going through chaos*, but if there was, I couldn't put my finger on it. Wondering if I needed a spiritual infusion, I tried to go to the local Catholic church a couple of times, but I felt nothing.

I enjoyed the weeks that the girls were with me. When I was alone in the house, the days dragged on and the nights were endless. I re-decorated and painted the house. I read books and watched movies. I went back to salsa dancing and contemplated getting back into it professionally again. But I couldn't stomach anything related to romance.

I met a man who was very keen on competing in dance and wanted me as his partner, so we trained. The challenge for me was that I was a 30-something single mother with a mortgage, and I was competing against 20-somethings who could devote all of their time and energy into dance. Then there the fact that my hip would cause me agony after dancing, but I kept trying to pretend there was no problem. I went for hip injections that helped me move, but the fact remained that I needed a hip replacement, and I did not want to accept that.

2 - 3 Tears

My dance partner was about 10 years older than me, and he had no kids, so he did not understand that I was not always available. This eventually became a problem for him, and though our dancing was quite exceptional, we parted ways because I could not devote the time to it that was required. If I was living some other life, a life where I was rich and free, I would have just quit my day job and danced—but alas, that was not in the cards for me. I still held out hope that surgery would allow me to get back into dancing, but for the moment I had to let go of that dream, which was a little was tough and made me sad.

Stripped of that particular passion, loneliness and the desire to be loved crept in again and took over. Four or five months after Brian and I separated, I began browsing on a dating website, and I met Pat right away. Pat was not handsome in a conventional way, but he had angular features, tanned Mediterranean skin and impossibly long eyelashes framing beautiful brown eyes that seemed to pierce right into my soul. While the combination attracted me, there was something about him that made me feel uneasy, so I kept him at arm's length for a while, casually dating him while I dated others.

Soon, however, he became more of a fixture in my life. He became very attentive, which I began to welcome. He would bring me flowers and make me mixed CDs, things that Brian had never done. He also told me how beautiful I was, and was incredibly romantic. He would cook dinner, complete with candlelight and music, and we would dance in the living room afterward. Sometimes I would wake up and go out to my car in the morning to find all the snow cleared off, and a poem or note on the windshield, a kindness he would do on his way to work in the early morning hours.

Soon, I stopped seeing other men. While I had only been marginally attracted to him at first, because he was the first man I'd met who was so deeply enamored with me, I thought I could learn to love him. He was easy to talk with, and was an attentive listener.

We spoke for hours about God and the universe, and how we are all connected. I felt a spiritual connection with him that I had never felt before with a man. He said and did all the 'right' things to win me over, and before long I thought I had finally found my prince. He grew more handsome to me, and I began to trust him.

There was no doubt he had deep feelings for me; the first time he cried in front of me he told me he was shedding tears of happiness, because I made him feel special. I thought it was touching for him to be so emotionally vulnerable. His tears were because he loved me so much, and part of me melted. It made me want to open up to him more.

However, it started getting a little odd when he would cry and say how sad he was that he always had to pack an overnight bag and stay over for a couple of days, and how he wished he didn't have to unpack and repeat the cycle over and over. He said when he left me, he missed me too much, and that he wanted us to be together all of the time. While part of me liked the idea of someone being so in love with me, on principle alone I did not want to live with him just yet. There was something about him I could not put my finger on that didn't sit right with me. I could not, in good conscience, dive headfirst into a shared living arrangement with him and put my hard-won security at risk.

Four months after we started dating, Pat got into a bad car accident and suffered a pretty bad concussion. My gears switched into helper mode, and I was pleased on some level that my medical training could be useful once again. Pat's family lived far away, so I told him to come and stay with me while he recovered, because it was obvious he could not take care of himself. I nursed his wounds and cared for him, while the days turned into weeks. Of course the intimacy of this new arrangement escalated his feeling for me; he said he wanted to marry me one day, and that there was no point paying for two separate dwellings.

While he was not completely wrong, something still didn't feel right for me and I resisted, which made him cry. He said he was *so* hurt, and said that I didn't really love him the way he loved me.... and I caved. He officially moved in.

For a while, things were good and I started to get used to him being around. His kids came over on weekends and got along really well with my girls, so I started to think that maybe we could be a big happy family.

A few months later, my dad, my girls and I went to Austria to visit family. Pat was a little pouty about me going away and leaving him behind, but this trip had been planned long before we'd gotten serious, and it was something I really wanted to do. Austria always tugged at my heartstrings, and I had fond memories of the time I spent there during my childhood and how happy I'd been. I wanted to share that with my children. I also knew my aging father longed to see his family one last time, but that he was in no shape to go on his own.

The trip was great. We spent two weeks visiting family and sightseeing, and I felt so much peace. I barely thought of Pat at all, which struck me as odd, but I was just so happy spending time with my daughters and getting in touch with our heritage. One of my goals was to take a cable car up a mountain. We tried a few times, but rain ruined our plans. As this was one important thing on my trip to-do list, I felt compelled to keep trying.

I'm so glad I insisted. One of the happiest moments of my life was when we got off that cable car, walked towards the clouds and then, when we reached the top of the mountain, found ourselves overlooking a countryside of vibrant, green, rugged terrain and snow-capped mountains. The world came to an abrupt halt. Tears streamed down my face and I almost fell to my knees at the captivating beauty of what I beheld.

It was almost too much to take in, and yet I didn't even blink for fear of missing even one second. My soul felt as if it were floating in the clouds, light as a feather. At this moment, I came to know what contentment felt like. It transcended words. I imagined Heaven felt like this, and I did not want to leave. Now, years later, when times are tough I go back there in my mind. It still touches and moves me deeply. I have never been able to physically re-visit that place, but oh how my heart yearns for it. There was a time, in my early teens, that I dreamt about moving there. If there is such a thing as a parallel universe, I am definitely living in the Austrian mountains. A part of my heart will always be in Austria.

The rest of the trip flew by, filled with spending precious moments with my girls at the spa, eating tons of strudel, and seeing my dad so happy to be with his family and his childhood friends.

Not too long after we arrived home, and about eight months into our relationship, Pat and I started to argue—or at least *he* did. He would suddenly get intensely angry at the smallest things that I did or said. It started small enough, but then these arguments got longer and longer and much of what he said did not make sense to me.

In my previous relationships, I was never one to argue, and I generally tried to avoid conflict as much as possible, so this was new territory. I was so used to the 'silent treatment' that I did not know how to fight. I was like a deer in the headlights when he would yell. I remember one fight we had when he found old pictures of me dancing with other men on my Facebook page. He'd known I had danced professionally for years from the day we met—and of *course* I would have pictures of that! However, when I pointed that out to him, he got defensive and his anger soared. He literally kept me up all night until I agreed to delete the pictures, and even after I did, he kept yelling and pacing around the room.

His anger scared me but it passed, and the next day he apologized and said he only acted that way because he loved me so much. I felt a little apprehensive about his excuse, but he was back to his loving self so I buried my feelings. But the problem didn't go away. In fact, the fights began to escalate each time they happened. In the heat of the argument, he would bring up old issues I thought we had already resolved, over and over again. I learned quickly not to answer back, as it seemed only to fuel his anger, but with each fight, I became more and more frightened of him. He would literally yell at me for hours, with so much rage, while I sat quietly. Because this was not the Pat I knew, I thought that maybe these angry outbursts were because of his head injury, so I persevered with the relationship.

During this time, I was experiencing a lot of hip pain and had been going every six months for injections into my hip joint. They were a little painful at first, but after a few days, they worked like magic. My doctor told me that soon, however, they would stop working and that surgery was imminent. By now my other knee had started giving me problems, so I had another arthroscopic surgery on that knee. They fixed up the torn cartilage, but told me the primary problem was my hip, which was causing the knee pain. They said my knee problems would not go away until I had my hip replaced.

By late that summer, things with Pat seemed to be on the upswing and I felt good. I opened my heart to him and we began sharing our life stories in great detail with one another, including painful memories from our pasts. I think one of the things that made me fall in love with him was that he gave me undivided attention, soaking up every word I said with real interest. It felt good to be with someone who was intent on knowing who I was. I found that I still had to walk on eggshells around him sometimes, mostly when I could sense his mood being off, but he was very helpful around the house and we laughed a lot.

One day we were all driving up to my dad's old cottage for the weekend. I was feeling pretty happy, when suddenly I felt my heart stop and then a few seconds later re-start. The heartbeat was so strong that I felt it in my neck and my head—and it even caused me to lose my breath for a second. It did this every other heartbeat for a couple of minutes, and then it went away. I chalked it up to being a strange, random things and continued with my weekend. By Sunday, however, it had started again and this time it persisted for a few hours. I kept feeling my heart stop and restart with a thud like a crack of thunder. Something was not right.

It was scary, but because my kids were with us, I didn't say anything as I did not want to worry them. However, eventually I became so dizzy and weak that I decided to go to the hospital. Pat and I left the cottage, while Juan came to pick up the girls.

The doctor did some tests and they let me go home after referring me to a cardiologist. I had more tests, but no one could figure out what was going on. Meanwhile, the skipping heartbeats kept me up at night, making me very tired during the day. Sometimes, I would be out walking and have to stop and sit on the sidewalk to rest, because I'd get so dizzy I thought I would pass out. Various doctors tried different medications on me, and the side effects generally left me feeling worse. I was told I needed heart surgery. They planned to do a 'cardiac ablation', a procedure that burns tissue in your heart to block abnormal electrical signals and restore a normal heart rhythm. The procedure involved inserting a catheter through my groin to my heart. I tried to convince myself it was no big deal but a small part of me was scared.

Within a couple of weeks, I was lying on the operating room table, being sedated. My eyes closed and I began to drift off. Suddenly in the background, I heard voices saying, "We're losing her."

I tried to open my eyes, but I couldn't. Shortly after that I woke up, still on the operating table. The doctors told that they had to reverse the sedation and medications because my heart couldn't handle it and my heart rate had plummeted dangerously low. "Stay very still," I was told. And then they told me that they would have to do the procedure with no sedation or medication.

I agreed to lie completely still, and did so, even when I felt wires wiggle their way through my chest. Then, four hours into the procedure, they had mapped out the spots to burn out—but the machine broke. The doctor told me that it was the first time in ten years that this had ever happened.

Over the next two hours they tried two more catheters ... and when the doctor told me they would have to stop and try again in a few days, I could not hold back my tears. I had been perfectly still on an operating room table, fully awake, for six hours. My back was stiff, my hip hurt, and I wanted to scream—and yet the reward for my efforts was to return in a few days to do it all over again.

Pat was so kind and sweet, and he never left my side. He slept on the hospital floor next to me, and the nurses were touched at how devoted he was. I was told I had to lay still on my back for yet another six hours. During that terrible time, I thought I couldn't have found a more loving, concerned partner. All of his anger issues were forgotten. If someone could sleep on a dirty hospital floor just to comfort me, he was worth keeping.

Less than a week later I was back in surgery. Again, they could use no sedation or medication on me, but this time it only took four hours, and they got the right spots. It was a very strange sensation to feel pieces of my heart being burned. Pat once again spent the night on the floor next to my bed, and I went home the next day. It took some time for me to recover—I would get very winded and tired doing the simplest thing—but I kept pushing myself and, within a few months, I was back to normal. I went on to have occasional episodes of skipped beats, but they eventually disappeared.

A few weeks after my surgery, I went for a very slow-paced walk around the block to visit my brother, who was living with my dad at the time. He'd never called me to ask how I was doing after my heart surgery and it hurt my feelings, because we had become quite close in the past two years. And then, when I told him the story of my surgery, he barely heard a word. He just said, "You're okay now, right?"

I chalked his lack of response up to the fact that he was always stoned, and also that he was depressed and having trouble with his Crohn's disease, and so instead of telling him how I felt, I offered to help take him to the doctor. He refused, and changed the subject to our father. We were both very concerned about Dad because it seemed like he was being taken advantage of by a renovations contractor. The costs seemed extraordinarily high for what was being done, and we tried to talk to him about it, but he wouldn't listen. We would get him to promise that he would have any more work to the house without talking to us first, but a few days later the contractors would be back doing more work. It was frustrating, and Nick was reaching the end of his patience with dad's stubbornness, as was I. He said he would have a talk with the contractor, but it never happened. I wondered if I should get involved, but I didn't have the energy to pursue it.

I knew my brother Nick was really troubled, though he didn't seem to want to talk about it much. To encourage him to lean on me emotionally, I invited him over, or went to visit him, quite often. He would really light up when he played with my children ... but then he would return to a detached state when the fun was over.

One day, Nick and I stood outside my house and he told me that his Crohn's disease had gotten quite bad. He said that if it got any worse, and he had to get a colostomy, that he would rather die. Then he told me that one day he would just go off into the bushes and we'd never see him again.

Frightened at his words, I told him how much we all loved him that I would find him a good doctor and go with him to the appointment. Then I reminded him of a conversation we'd once had when I found out my ex-boyfriend, Earl, had committed suicide. Both of us had been saddened, and Nick had flat out told me he would never want to cause that kind of pain to his family. After reminding him of his words, I tried to cheer him up and offered to set him up with one of my friends, but he refused. However, by the end of the conversation, he seemed happier and was smiling, and so I thought I'd made him feel better, and that things would be okay.

Nick

One day in early June, about four and a half months after my heart surgery, I was walking around the block and saw Nick's car turn a corner in the distance. I felt a strange yearning to wave my arms and yell and make him stop so that I could hug him, but he never saw me and I was too far away. A few hours later I got a text saying how he would always love me and the girls, and that I had been the best sister.

When I read it, a sense of panic filled me. I ran as fast as my feet could carry me over to his house. No one was home, so I let myself in and went up the stairs into his bedroom. I found the suicide note on his desk. My mind went hazy and I tried to call him, but the phone went straight to voicemail. I texted him to tell him that I loved him, and to call me. He just *couldn't* be gone. His note ended in a happy face telling me that I could have his car. Who puts a happy face on a suicide note?

Deep down I knew he was gone, but I didn't want to believe it, so I told myself that maybe he really wasn't—that maybe there was still a chance he was alive. *No,* I thought. *This just can't be real.* I sat on his bed wondering what to do next. The call from the police confirming his death came only moments later. My dear, sweet brother Nick had put a shotgun in his mouth, pulled the trigger and was now dead.

The world went black and fuzzy. I don't remember how I got home, but I remember collapsing on the floor of my front hallway in heaving sobs. Pat came rushing to my side, but I couldn't speak. All I could manage to get out between breaths was, "Nick is dead." 'My Nicky' as I used to call him when we were kids, was no more. I could no longer look into his bright blue eyes or laugh with him. I couldn't go over to his house for a smoke with him. He would miss out on his nieces growing up. My birthday party was a few days away and he'd said he would be there for it! I couldn't fathom a world without my baby brother in it.

Pat called my parents and invited them over as I got up and tried to pull myself together. I had to turn off the unbearable pain and detach from it, it was the only way. One of the hardest things I have ever had to do in my life was to tell my parents that their son was dead—and not just by some freak accident; I had to tell my mom and dad that their one and only son had killed himself.

The gut-wrenching wails from my mother, and seeing my father in tears for the first time in my life, broke me—but I couldn't show it, because they needed me. I sent Pat out to buy a pack of cigarettes while my parents and I waited for the police to come. I think that until the police came, there was a part of my mom and dad that didn't believe it had really happened.

I sat chain-smoking as the officer told us about his death. True to his words months earlier, he had gone far up north out to the bushes alone to do it. His death had been instantaneous and apparently I was the last person he'd messaged. He'd called 911 right after he texted me, and then shut off his phone.

The next worst thing I've ever had to do was to identify the body of my little brother after he'd died such a violent death. I had seen all kinds of gruesome things as a paramedic, but none of it had been inflicted on someone I loved so dearly. I wanted to just bury myself under the covers and cry for a week, but I couldn't. I had to be the rock for my parents, who were barely coping. Meanwhile, Pat was so supportive during everything, and worked for two days straight without sleep to make a beautiful video tribute to Nick for the funeral.

It was an incredibly difficult time. Family and friends could not grasp why such a handsome, kind, young man would take his own life. However, I understood it. I had been in that dark spot, and if I'd had access to guns as he did, I probably would have done the same. I knew that once that darkness overtakes a soul, there is no stopping the urge to attempt suicide. I'd gotten lucky and survived those urges, but Nick had not.

Looking back, I believe my brother was an empath who could not handle the intense emotions he felt. Instead, he buried them by smoking pot. Nick was the kind of man who would drop everything to help someone in need, but he was very private about his feelings and he had trouble opening up. He was such a good, kind soul that the atrocities and crimes in our world would eat at him. He could not fathom how people could be so cruel to one another, and subsequently he struggled with depression most of his life. I knew his pain and how he came to that point. We had grown up in the same household. Our core subconscious feelings of longing to loved and accepted were similar; however, we had different coping mechanisms—Nick remained single and turned to drugs, while I filled my life with a string of toxic relationships.

Maybe, I thought, *if I had been open with him about my own experiences, and suggested he try therapy like I did, it might have made a difference.* I knew what it felt like to have overpowering darkness wash over me like a tidal wave. But then again, he may not have been interested in talking to anyone about his feelings. Nick wore a mask that was even thicker than mine and would not let anyone in. Both of us were similarly emotionally cut off from ourselves, and lacked awareness of the darkness that swam through us.

Nick did not leave a will, and there was some debt. There were a lot of meetings with banks and lawyers that I hobbled to with my cane, because my hip pain was getting worse. I tried to stay strong, and never told my parents the aftermath and work I had to deal with, because they were going through enough grief.

Going through Nick's things tore at my heart. A couple of his friends came over to help, and the positive side of this experience was that I got to know a different side of Nick as they shared some of their memories of him. However, when I was alone I felt angry with Nick—angry that he'd left me with a heavy burden of work; angry that I was alone to look after my parents as they aged; furious that my children would never get to know their only uncle.; angry at him for lying about coming to my birthday party.

As selfish as it sounds, I was enraged that my birthday would now be marked forever by his death, and what made it worse was that I couldn't tell anyone how angry I was because I was afraid of what people would think. Eventually the anger died down and changed to feelings of guilt for my own responses. Feeling guilty was almost as debilitating as feeling angry. It lasted a few months, and brought up such uncomfortable thoughts as, *could I have stopped him if I was a better, more attentive sister? What if I had taken him more seriously when he told me of his plans to 'disappear' those months ago?*

After a while, I realized that this kind of thinking would not bring him back, and was only destroying me. I had my children and my parents to be there for. I worked hard on focusing on the good memories of the times we had shared, but it was hard to get the last time I saw him, lying dead in the morgue, out of my head.

The biggest thing that brought me peace over losing my brother was that I knew, without a shadow of a doubt, that I would see him again in Heaven. Despite early Catholic lessons that taught us a person would burn in Hell if he or she took their own life, I believed God was merciful and loving, that he would understand Nick to be in so much pain that he needed to return home, and that He would welcome him with loving arms.

Pat 2.0

As life went on, and I tried to recover as best I could from Nick's death, things with Pat started to get rocky again, and his mood swings became more erratic and intense. He never returned to work after his accident, and he began to sit home all day long while I worked. At times he would help out with house chores, but at other times he did nothing but play on his computer.

I was not happy about the situation because, in my eyes, he definitely had the capabilities to work. At my urging, he got a part-time job, but he just didn't want to work and he soon found an excuse to quit. I stayed quiet. I was still dealing with my grief and the intense pain in my hip every day, and the opioid painkillers kept me in a detached state, but the truth was that it often felt like I was parenting three children, instead of two.

The silver lining during this time is that my father and I began mending our relationship, and he started opening up to me a little about his life. One day I went to visit my dad, and I caught him in a moment when he was feeling very depressed about his divorce and the death of my brother. He spoke very candidly to me that day. He said that *he* had brought on everything bad that had happened in our family, and that everything was all his fault. He said it was *his* fault his wife had left him; it was *his* fault that he had a son who committed suicide; and, that it was *his* fault that he had a daughter who couldn't keep a man, and who'd been whoring around.

I was caught off guard, and so I sat down, dug my fingernails into the palms of my clenched fists to keep my defensiveness from getting the better of me, and asked him why he felt this way.

The air in the room seemed to thicken and go still as Dad told me his story. He started by saying that he had waited a long time to get married, and hadn't thought it would ever happen. He'd met my mother at work, fallen in love with her at first sight, and struggled with the fact that she was not interested. At that time, he told me, he was involved in a cult of sorts. He'd been lured into it thinking it would further his spiritual journey and belief in God; however, the group was not what he expected. Instead, they were interested in transcendental meditation, astral travel, and invoking spirits—but he did not elaborate further.

I could tell there was a lot more he was not telling me, but I did not question him; instead, I just sat in silence and waited for him to talk. Finally, he continued, saying that far from what he had hoped for, this group was in fact very *far* from God.

The intensity with which he said this sparked a childhood memory for me. I suddenly recalled Dad being fiercely adamant in telling my brother and I that we were to never open a particular green suitcase he had stored in the crawlspace. He impressed upon us that when he died, men would show up at the door to collect the books in that suitcase—and that we were to hand them over without question. His words scared me, and yet on more than one occasion I opened that green suitcase anyway ... and then I would quickly close it for fear of getting caught. However, when I was a teenager, curiosity finally got the better of me and with great trepidation, I opened the suitcase to delve deeper. It was filled with a bunch of thin, dusty books. I opened one, and I remember seeing some kind of instruction on ritual, and some weird spells. The books suddenly felt like thick black poison in my hands. Scared, I put them away and never touched them again.

I sat listening intently to my father as he went on to tell me that, because my mother was not interested in dating him, he invoked a demon to get her to fall in love with him. It worked; she fell in love with him and they got married. Then he told me that, around the time I was 13 years old, he heard God speak to him, telling him he'd taken the wrong path. He told me he fell to his knees sobbing, and became a fervent Catholic after that. He also told me he knew he would have to pay for all the wrongs he had done ... and that this was the reason all the bad things that had happened in our family.

I sat there speechless, unsure of how to respond to what I had just heard. Thoughts raced through my head like pieces of a puzzle coming together, such as how he'd called me 'heathen' or 'devil's child' in my youth—which now made sense. *Was I really the sum of demonic incantations?* I thought about how I was always terrified of going into the basement in our home, because there seemed to be a dark presence there. I literally could *not* go down there; I was convinced that I would die, or get swallowed up in blackness. The basement was where my father sometimes held meetings, and my mother had spoken of a dark presence in the house for years, saying that she sometimes felt the air change in her bedroom, followed by a dark presence sitting on the end of her bed. Was a demon following my family around? Or was God punishing my father, as he believed?

Once, when I was about 19 and still dating Shane, he mentioned that something in the basement scared him, like a ghost. An atheist, Shane was definitely not the type to make up that kind of thing. We were alone in my parent's house while they were away in Europe, and decided to investigate. We went into the basement and opened the door to my dad's room where he had sometimes held his cult meetings—and Shane was knocked backward. He fell to the ground and turned completely white, the hairs standing up on his arms, while I felt a bitterly cold wind pass through me, and some intense nausea. Shane said a spirit had passed through us, and it wasn't a good one ... and while my logical brain had a hard time believing it, I'd felt it too.

Now, after hearing my father's confession, I started thinking more deeply about my past. As kids, when my dad had yelled at us I'd always thought it was more than just a father yelling at his children. The enraged person had been my dad, but also *not* my dad. In retrospect, it seemed as if a powerful dark presence had been behind his rage—and the powerlessness it had invoked in me as a child had been terrifying.

I looked at my father, confused. I didn't know what to make of all I had just heard. It was disturbing and I felt like I'd entered the proverbial twilight zone. Was I under some sort of evil demonic curse? Was I possessed? Is this why I had so many problems? I did not want to acknowledge or even think about the fact that I had felt something dark following me around all my life. Or that maybe it was still there.

I pushed all I'd heard aside. In retrospect, I know it was because I was too scared to delve into it any deeper. What scared me even more was that when Pat yelled at me, I felt that same darkness come from behind *him*—and I felt powerless against it.

I got up to leave my dad's place and decided to focus on the fact that he had made a remarkable change in his life, and was a completely different man than the one he had been in my childhood. As I left, I felt bad for him because he was consumed with heavy guilt and I tried to console him, but he said that it was his cross to carry and that he never wanted to speak of it again.

I was scheduled to have a hip replacement by December of that year. The doctors told me there was nothing left of my hip; it was just bone on bone. I was not even nervous about the surgery; I just wanted the pain to stop, and to be able to walk again. The pain had become unbearable, and the injections and medications were no longer working. I had waited long enough. I was only thirty-eight years old.

The day of the surgery, Pat came with me to the hospital, but he was acting quite odd and hyper. By this time in our relationship, he was starting to get stoned regularly to the point that conversations with him were useless, so he was not really a support for me.

I woke up from the surgery in the recovery room to pain so strong in my in my newly-operated-upon hip that I'd never felt anything like it in my life. Apparently, the hip dislocated when they transferred me from one bed to another, and the shiny, new hip had dislocated and come through my groin. I remember the doctor trying to pull it back into place. I passed out from the pain.

They took me back into the operating room and fixed it, making the immense pain subside somewhat. Because they usually try to have patients up and trying to walk the day after a hip replacement, the next day the nurse came in to get me up. That was when I realized that I had no feeling at all in my leg. Suddenly, I had a team of doctors and specialists hovering around me poking and prodding and doing tests.

The prognosis was not good. The doctors told me that it was likely I would never be able to use that leg again, because there was nerve damage. I remember lying in the hospital bed after hearing this news and feeling so alone, sad and hopeless. I had no one to reassure me because at this point my parents had left my bedside, because they didn't exactly like Pat, while Pat, who was stoned out of his mind, had taken off and was trying to hit on a friend of mine who'd been visiting.

I wondered, *how can it be that I will never walk again?* It had been hard to give up running, followed by dancing … but to give up *walking*? There was no way I would accept that. I simply would not accept that ridiculous diagnosis! I was determined to recover, to walk again, and to prove them wrong. It would be a long road to recovery, but there was no way I was going to accept a fate of not being able to walk while my girls needed me—and while I was living with a man I was becoming increasingly fearful of.

When I got home from the hospital I was feeling cautiously optimistic because, while my leg was still quite numb, some feeling had come back to the point where I could use a walker. The doctors told me there was not *total* nerve damage, like they'd originally thought, and that with time and hard work there was a chance I would be able to walk almost normally again. I was more determined than that; I planned to not only walk again, but dance.

Recovery, however, was exhausting and terribly lonely. Most people in my age range were still fit, active and a long way from hip surgery. It was generally a procedure associated with an older crowd, so no one knew what to say to me. Meanwhile, my supposed partner Pat was battling his own moods, and trying out new medications.

One of the worst days of my life happened a few days after I got home. That ill-fated time that was supposed to be joyous—but instead, Pat went into a full-blown manic episode. I don't recall what started it, but I was lying in bed, doped up on pain medication ... and the next thing I remember, he was standing over me, yelling and threatening me that he would make it so I would lose my job, and my kids would be taken away from me. He said he had called my mother and told her how concerned he was about me taking so many pills, and that my mother told him I was a junkie and had *always* taken too many pills. He threatened that he would make it so I had no one in my life, and that he would turn my entire family against me. He yelled something about me not appreciating how he had gone to great lengths to set up my room for me and take care of me. Then he threatened to kill himself.

I didn't quite catch it all, and none of it was making sense—but with his near genius IQ and computer skills, I had no doubt he could pull this off.

Thank goodness my kids were with their father that week. I thought he was going to hit me as he hovered above me, his fist raised. He was filled with such rage, and I got so scared, that I called the police. I could not have him around me after all I'd just gone through. The stress was too much.

The police arrived and, as I lay in bed, I thought for sure they would see the state he was in and commit him to the psych ward. But the most bizarre thing happened: He spoke to them completely and utterly normally, as if nothing had happened at all! I lay in bed listening to him tell the police he was glad I'd called them, because he was worried that I was suicidal. Then an officer came in and spoke to me. I explained everything that had happened and they told me that because he appeared stable, and there was no assault, they couldn't do anything. However, I could ask him to leave my home, since he did not own it. I immediately told them to remove him from the premises, and that he was unwelcome in my home. At that point, I did not care whether or not they believed my story or not—I just wanted Pat gone.

Alone in the house and unable to do much of anything for myself, I found a new resolve and strength that I did not know I had. My mother occasionally came to change my sheets and bring food, but I didn't want her to help more than that, because I didn't want them to find out what had happened with Pat.

When she was around, pretending everything was okay became too exhausting. My mother can be dramatic, and is a constant worrier, so I couldn't show her my pain. Besides, she was still mourning my brother ... and then there was the fact that she had called me a pill popper which, when I questioned her about it, she brushed it off. All in all, it was easier just to recover on my own.

I also didn't want anyone else to see me struggle. It would have been embarrassing to let anyone see how hard I had to work just to get to the bathroom with my walker and get myself onto the toilet. Getting back up off the toilet was even worse; it took all my strength and energy, yet I persevered because I did not want to be dependent on anyone. In fact, I was so determined to do this on my own that I stopped taking my pain medication, as it made me feel dopey and I needed my wits about me to get through this.

I had a nurse come in a few times a week, and a physiotherapist. They both said the only way my hip could have dislocated anteriorly was if it had been dropped off the table. This made sense, though the hospital never admitted to it. Some people tried to encourage me to pursue this legally, but I just didn't have it in me. All I wanted to do was to get better. It would take a lot of hard work and perseverance, but what choice did I have?

My kids were my strength, and knowing they depended on me filled me with a strength that did not feel like my own. I went to all kinds of therapies and diligently did my exercises at home. Little by little I got stronger, and within four months I only needed a cane to walk. I would end up always walking with a limp because they had to make my leg longer during surgery, and the nerve damage would never completely go away but I was still determined. People constantly told me how strong and positive I was, and how much I inspired them, but inside I didn't feel happy or positive. I was just doing what I had to do, and going through the motions. I tried hard not to think about what had happened with Pat, because if I started crying, I knew I would not be able to stop … and I needed to focus.

A couple of months later, Pat and I started talking again and told me that he had been diagnosed with bipolar disorder. According to the doctors, the car accident had ignited it. He said he was getting help, and that the manic episode he'd had after my surgery was due to an antidepressant that didn't mix well with marijuana and bipolar disorder, and had induced his mania. He said that he had a disease no different than my arthritis, that it was not something he had asked for. He asked me to believe that he was still the same guy I once loved. Then he cried, apologized and promised that his new medication was working, and it would never happen again.

We talked and visited, since he was in an apartment nearby, and bit by bit he won me over again with his magnetic charm, attention, promises, and romance. He told me he would never, ever hurt me, and that I knew as well as he did that we were soul mates and were meant to be together. I'm not sure why I caved.

Maybe it was because I was just feeling tired and vulnerable, and thought that with my health issues I would never find someone to love me. Maybe it was his rationalization that we both had diseases we didn't ask for and deserved to be happy. Maybe I felt sorry for him because the accident was not his fault, and I remembered the kind, romantic man I had first met who was still there somewhere. Whatever it was, I convinced myself that he would get better with enough love and support.

I was wrong. Instead, our relationship went back and forth, up and down as he bounced between mania and depression. Entire walls got punched through. I got called every vulgar name imaginable. Vases were thrown at my head. Furniture was smashed. New promising medications and therapy were tried. In between, there were apologies, tears, laughter, long talks, and romance. He moved in and out several times.

His manic highs were magnetic, in a way. He was so much fun to be with, and we would have long insightful conversations on life, God and spirituality. On the highs, he played silly games with the kids and all seemed well. Days and weeks would go by when he was his charming 'normal' self ... and then the depression would come like clouds on a windy day. Then, he would cry for hours and bury himself on the couch, hoping to die.

I tried so hard to lift his spirits but nothing worked. He had very rapid cycling bipolar, and so I never knew from one moment to the next what would happen. I continued to hold onto the belief that he would get better, and that things would go back to how they once were. Ultimately, I loved and I hated him at the same time. The love was for the kind, sweet person I knew was buried inside; the hate was for the 'Mr. Hyde' who came out at the bad times. I felt that I had to show compassion because he, like me, was suffering. I enjoyed the happy 'in-between' times, which recharged my batteries.

One day, Pat had another bad manic episode, a terrifying one. While manic, he took out a butcher knife, held it up, and told me he was going to slice his own arm open and then put the knife in my hands and tell everyone that I had tried to kill him.

I was terrified. His eyes held so much hatred that I had no doubt he would come at me if I said one word. He was a very strong, muscular man in those days, physically intimidating. To calm him down, I tried to tell him I loved him, while my heart was racing in fear. He put the knife down, thank God, but continued screaming and yelling. This went on for hours. I remember being on the floor, curled up in a ball with my head in my hands, crying in terror while he uttered the most horrifying threats imaginable. Eventually I got up and tried to get away from him, but he followed me around the house yelling incessantly. He even pushed me into a wall.

Suddenly he got a phone call, and he began speaking like there was absolutely nothing going on. He sounded like a regular, happy guy. I had witnessed this dramatic change in personality before, but it never ceased to shock me how he could just turn his craziness off and on. I felt like I was in a horror movie; it did not seem real.

While he was still talking, I seized my opportunity and ran out of the house. I hid in a neighbor's yard and called the police, because all I knew was that I had to get away from him because I knew things would end badly. I was trembling in fear, and utterly humiliated to be crouched down in the mud between some bushes, in someone else's yard. Nobody in my life knew about what was going on in the relationship, because I was filled with shame and fear. How could I have let this happen? I was an educated woman with a respectable career. I had children! Just how had I ended up here?

Once again, the police came and took him away. It took hours before I stopped trembling, and the only saving grace was that my kids were at their fathers' that week and did not witness it. In fact, by the grace of God, they never really experienced *any* of Pat's intense episodes. He seemed to save it for when we were alone.

Months later, like a dog goes back to eat it's own vomit, I opened myself up to Pat yet again. He knew a gullible sugar mama when he saw one, and he knew all the right words to say. He told me that after the police had taken him away, he'd spent some time in the psych ward and was now on medication and seeing a psychiatrist. He insisted he had changed.

Pretty stupid of me to take him back, right? But I was convinced Pat was worthy of love and compassion and that, just because he had a mental illness, it didn't mean he was *less* worthy. After all, he couldn't control it—or so he said. The truth was that I was so broken on the inside that I had no hope left in me. After all my pain and surgeries, and the loss of my brother, I did not have any emotional strength left in me to fight him. I felt utterly worthless on the inside and I believed I didn't deserve to be treated well. When he said I would never find anyone else who would love me as much as he did, I believed him.

It was around that time that I became even *more* detached from my feelings. I guess I believed that if I could pretend none of the bad stuff had happened, then it hadn't. Maybe I was reacting out of fear, or maybe I thought he really *had* changed.

Once again, things went smoothly for a while. Throughout our relationship, the good times were so incredible, that I wanted them back. He would throw me enough little scraps of romance and tenderness that I would believe he was still the loving man I had originally met. But things gradually started to go downhill. First, Pat stopped taking his medication; then, his moods began to shift. I began to get more and more distant from him, and he began to pull away too. I was too scared to break up with him, as I believed he would make good on all his threats. He'd told me that if I ever left him he would kill himself, but that before he did he would ruin me. He was an expert at computer hacking, so I did not doubt that he capable of this.

I was under an incredible amount of stress and so, at the end of my rope, I began to pray. I had not prayed very much in my life up until then, but now I prayed fervently every night for God to take him out of my life. I begged and pleaded. Living with him had become so stressful, I felt like I had no way out. I had lost so much weight from my already thin frame, that friends and family began expressing concern. I felt nauseous and on edge all the time; however I told everyone that I was happy, and not to worry. I was not ready to face up to the fact that I had allowed this man into my life, not once but multiple times. I felt dead inside.

Healthwise, as I had been having pain in my foot, I finally went to have it checked out. The surgeon said my foot was severely arthritic and that she needed to fuse the bone in my foot with a metal plate. Pat came with me to the surgery, but during my two-month long recovery, he was moody. We were becoming more and more distant from each other, and I felt like I had to walk on eggshells around him. All the long talks we used to like to have were long over; now, he was going out more and more, pretending to be looking for work. I knew he was lying, but I was glad to have a few hours away from him.

One night Pat came in quite late and fell asleep on the couch. I had an urge to check his cell phone, something I'd not done in any previous relationship. I found texts from a woman he had been dating behind my back. While he was still asleep, I texted her, pretending to be him. I told this woman (while pretending to be him), that I had just broken up with my girlfriend and asked if I could come to stay with her, right away. She said 'yes'.

I woke him up, showed him the phone and told him that his girlfriend was expecting him, and he had 15 minutes to get out of my life. He left, throwing all kinds of accusations, and telling me that I hadn't been a good wife anyway.

I knew it was over between him and I for good this time, but I didn't feel bad. It wasn't like I'd kicked him out into the cold with no money and nowhere to go … and while it hurt to know he'd cheated, I was relieved at the same time that God had provided me a way out. My prayers had been answered.

Pat 3.0

After Pat and I separated, there were a few days I spent alone in tears and misery, yet every day I managed to go to work and care for my children. A month later, I was back on the dating sites. Even as I write this, I see the absurdity in it. I was just so broken inside, and so lost.

Not knowing who I was without a man in my life, I signed up to meet the next charming prince who would save me. In retrospect, perhaps I also needed to distract myself from the wretched shame I felt for ever getting involved with Pat in the first place.

Eventually, after a few 'meet and greets', I met Brandon. We had a very nice coffee date that turned into dinner. He was attractive, extremely educated, and had a great job in the military, and he was divorced with no custody issues. We began seeing each other somewhat regularly, and I found him to be a decent man. He fell for me fast, taking me to hockey games and concerts in other cities, and wining and dining me at expensive restaurants I normally never would have dreamed of eating at. He also took me on a Caribbean vacation … and all this occurred within four months. I felt like a princess with him, and I really wanted to like him more than I did. He had an odd sense of humor, but he was harmless—and most importantly, I felt safe with him.

Meanwhile, ongoing back pain that had been with me for years was worsening. I'd always assumed my back issues were caused by injuries that had never healed from my paramedic days, but the pain kept getting worse and I began the round of doctors and tests. Eventually, one doctor told me I had joint hypermobility syndrome, and that all I needed was exercise. I had always been overly flexible, but this didn't feel like the answer to what was going on in my body, so I continued looking for answers.

Thinking that perhaps my back pain was related to my unresolved issues with Pat, I went back to counseling—but even to the therapist, I could not admit the full extent of how Pat had treated me. I played it down. The pain persisted. Eventually, I saw a top rheumatologist and *finally* I got an answer. He diagnosed me with ankylosing spondylitis, a condition I had never even heard of. It turned out that everything, from my heart issues to the arthritis in my foot and my hip replacement—not to mention the swelling and pain in my hands and fingers—were all related to this disease.

It was a relief to have a name for all this pain that had plagued me. Throughout my life, pain would come on out of the blue. One day, I would have back pain; then for the next few weeks my hands would swell up so much that I couldn't even open a door. Sometimes my knees would swell up and I could not navigate the stairs; other times my back and neck would be so sore I could barely turn my head, or even move. I'd ignored all of this as much as I could, because on other days I felt reasonably well. It was not lost on me that while I was with Pat and in constant fight or flight mode, the pain was as intrusive as usual, but now that I was with Brandon, who was very relaxed, I was feeling the pain more and more. I wondered if it had to do with no longer being in an adrenaline-fused state; maybe now that I no longer had adrenaline coursing through my veins on a daily basis, while waiting for the next fight, my body felt it was okay to let down its defenses.

It was around this time, roughly three and a half months into dating Brandon, that Pat got in touch. He started emailing me, saying he'd gotten help, done a lot of soul-searching, and was finishing school to be a reiki practitioner. He said he had spent a lot of time with a First Nations chief who had guided him, and that he had found his spiritual side. He said he missed me and wanted to see me again.

I resisted. I was skeptical that he had truly changed, so I didn't really engage, but I did send the occasional email back ... and in short order I realized that, despite everything that had happened, I was still in love with Pat. What I *didn't* realize, at least until much later, was that I was only in love with one *version* of him—the side that was fun, romantic and spiritual. I wanted to believe that was who he truly was, and I didn't want to believe all the bad stuff.

As soon as I acknowledged my feelings for Pat, I realized I was not being fair to Brandon, so I broke up with him. As wonderful as Brandon was, he also seemed quite materialistic, and I felt he wanted a barbie doll on his arm to attend his fancy functions more than a real relationship with *me*. He was broken-hearted when I told him, and I felt horrible, but within a few weeks, he'd already found someone new.

Pat and I continued to email back and forth, having deep conversations that revolved around God, purpose in life, love, and acceptance. These were the things that I had been searching for, and had even tried to find in a church at one time. I had often wondered, *why* can't *we all just be kind and love each other?* One month later I finally agreed to meet him.

When I saw Pat again, I realized right away that he was calmer than I had ever seen him. He really seemed to have become a new, improved version of the man I had known. He even looked different; what was once a toned, muscular body that he used to work hard on to keep 'pumped up' was now very slender; he sported a beard; and, the designer labels he'd been vain about had been replaced by casual clothing. Moreover, he seemed at peace.

He apologized to me for cheating, and then went on to explain that, because of his bipolar disorder, he had convinced himself that

I did not love him. He told me that soon after he left, he realized what he had done, and felt awful. He explained that the disorder caused him to create alternate realities that were very real to him, such as feeling like I didn't love him, but that he was healed now.

We had a good talk, and he really did seem better. He said he had found God, and that God had healed him by driving out a demon that had been the main cause for his anger. He spoke with such spiritual depth that it resonated with me, triggering the memory of what my dad had told me about his experience with the demonic. I wanted God to heal me too.

That day in the park, he got down on one knee and asked me to marry him. He said I was the only person ever who he'd ever truly loved, and that he would spend his life trying to make me happy and make up for all the wrongs he had done.

I didn't know what to say. I was in shock, so I told him I needed time to think about it. He seemed a little hurt, but covered it up really well and told me to take as much time as I needed. The man I had known six months before would have never given me that breathing room, so I started to really believe that he was better.

We began dating, but because he did not have a place to stay, he kind of invited himself to stay at my place. I didn't know how to say no to him, and so abandoning both logic and common sense, with mixed emotions I let him move in.

My kids had never seen his manic side, and so they welcomed him back. He had always been good to them and I am thankful they were spared all the bad stuff. For three weeks, things were absolutely magical with us. I bought a small trailer, and we went away on our first camping trip. We all had a really good time. Pat was relaxed, warm, and fun to be with, and I began seeing hope for the future.

We drove separate cars to get to the campsite, and I was the one towing the trailer behind my SUV. On the drive home, I had an impulse to turn down a certain road, to take an alternate route. The radio was blasting, the kids were singing and I ignored this feeling and took the highway anyway. It turned out that my decision would be life-altering, a pivotal moment—and a valuable life lesson about listening to my gut instincts.

As we pulled onto the highway, traffic came to an abrupt stop and I stopped along with almost everyone else. I say 'almost' because I remember hearing a loud 'bang' … and I don't remember much after that. Apparently, a BMW going 100 kilometres an hour rear-ended our trailer, bounced off, and went on to strike another vehicle. The trailer then jack-knifed and came through the driver's side of my car.

When I woke up, both my girls were crying and calling for me. I felt an awful pain in my head and face, and I had to spit out the glass that was in my mouth. I was dazed, and I remember thinking that we needed to get out of the car in case the propane tank on the trailer exploded. However, it seemed like everything was in a thick fog, and I had a hard time opening the door. All the windows were smashed in, and glass was absolutely everywhere. My youngest daughter was terrified and crying hysterically.

We managed to get out of the car and then we sat by the side of the highway and waited for the ambulance to come. My whole body hurt, especially my hip and my head, but all I could think of was my girls. I was not concerned with being treated myself; they needed me.

When the paramedics arrived, I remember them asking me a lot of questions. I told them what I knew, but for some reason I could not remember how old I was or what year it was. It was 2015 and I kept saying it was 1999. One look at our mangled car and it was obvious to the paramedics that I had to go to a trauma hospital, while my kids would be sent to another hospital to be checked out, as they seemed okay.

I was so upset that I could not be with them, but at the same time, my head was feeling fuzzy and painful, and I was growing more and more confused. I cried when I got to the hospital, because all I could think of was my girls and how I was not there for them. Juan had been called by the police, and he went to the hospital to be with them. I was grateful because, despite what had happened to our marriage, he was a good father.

It was only when looking back that I recalled that, just ten minutes before the accident, my youngest daughter—who was in the back seat on the driver's side—asked if she could lie down. This was something she had never done before. Not *ever*. My kids had never been ones to sleep in the car, but on this day, for some reason, she had asked to lay down. Thinking nothing of it in the moment, I let her, and so she lay down, placing her head on the passenger side seat. This likely saved her life; at the very least, it kept her from suffering serious injury, as the driver's side doors sustained the heaviest impact. This seemingly innocent request turned out to be absolutely remarkable. Many people would tell me that it was my brother's spirit that had protected her. I just thanked God that she listened to her instincts.

After much poking, prodding, testing, doctors confirmed that I had suffered a mild traumatic brain injury, a broken nose and significant soft tissue injury. I felt awful and, to make matters worse, my parents showed up while Pat was there, and they had a big fight with him in the emergency room. My mom couldn't stand Pat by then, and didn't want him near me. I couldn't believe they were fighting after what had just happened, so I asked my parents to leave. The rest of my stay in the hospital was hazy.

Recovering at home proved challenging. Since I'd had five or six prior concussions, my symptoms were intensely magnified. The headaches were horrific and half the time I never knew what I was doing. I was surrounded by paperwork for the insurance company, and even though I worked in the industry I had no clue how to fill them out. I pushed myself beyond limits and pretended to be okay so my girls would not be affected. They had luckily escaped with only minor aches that a few sessions of physiotherapy cured, but they were still shaken by the accident. I had to be strong for them. I also didn't want Pat to get stressed and go into mania. Although he hadn't wigged out on me since our reconciliation, I still did not trust him. Narcissists have a very hard time with these types of things.

I remember filling out forms and then, when I went to write my name, I couldn't remember how to spell it. I would go out and forget where I was. In the grocery store one day, I panicked because I could not remember how I had gotten there or what I was doing there in the first place. I couldn't remember my children's birth dates. I had trouble speaking and getting words out. I stuttered when I spoke, and people told me they had a hard time following me in conversation. However, fatigue proved to be the biggest challenge for me. It was unlike anything I had ever experienced. In my job, I heard people speak of fatigue associated with head injuries, but I had not really comprehended it until now. It was all consuming; it felt like lead weights were strapped to every joint of my body, and that I had not slept in a month, even though I practically did nothing *but* sleep. But no amount of sleep could quench this fatigue.

It would be a few months before my memory and speech, with therapy, began to improve; however, the headaches, brain fog and fatigue persisted. Still, I had no choice but to keep going and fighting to get better, so that's what I did.

My strategy in life has always been to fight hard. It's how I approached all my previous surgeries, relationships and life goals. When a doctor told me I would need three months to heal, I would aim to do it in *one* month. I would push through the pain and do my exercises diligently.

With my surgeries, this strategy paid off every single time—but this was a different beast I was facing. This time, it seemed like the harder I tried, especially in those first few months, the worse I got. An occupational therapist told me that I should have just stayed in a dark room for the first month to allow my brain to heal. It had never crossed my mind, even though I knew this too because in my job I specialized in head injury claims. Perhaps I was just too busy trying to get better to think of it, but even if someone had told me, with my stubbornness I doubt that I would have listened anyway.

I was finally referred to a brain injury clinic at the hospital, where I would continue to go for a full year. By this time I was starting to get irritable and impatient, and there were times that I felt sad for no reason at all. It was a frustrating to not have control over my own body, or my own emotions. I felt like I was going crazy, because I would forget things, especially when I was tired, and no matter how much I slept, I always felt exhausted. My brain felt like a scattered jigsaw puzzle that I could not piece together, and it upset me that I sometimes couldn't communicate what I wanted to say.

During this time, Pat reached his limit with his ability to provide compassion and care. Instead, he was constantly nagging at me, telling me that we needed a fresh start in a new house we should buy together, because the one we were in held too many bad memories for him. He said he was still trying to be a better person, but that he could not do it in that house. With my head the way it was, I could not even entertain such thoughts as what to cook for dinner, let alone moving. I told him we would have to wait until I felt better. His response was to take off for a few days, saying he needed to be in nature to meditate. I felt relieved when he left. I was beginning to feel like perhaps I shouldn't have gotten back together with him.

Pat came back from his nature break all aglow and apparently expected me to happily jump into his arms. I just couldn't. His not-so-subtle hints about moving, and about how he would be able to love me better in a new home were beginning to irritate me. He didn't have a penny to his name, and the house we lived in was in *my* name. Something in me knew I could not ever own anything with this man, let alone move somewhere with him. He had a dream of living in a remote location, far out of the city, and he tried to convince me how happy we would be in the country. I was not buying it. Looking back, I can see how it was a ploy to isolate me from my friends and family.

Once Pat realized that I would not sell my house and move out to the boonies, he had to come up with another plan. He wanted to start his own business but couldn't do it on his own. He told me he knew someone who was into natural healing, as he was, and who was interested in starting a business with him. The lady he wanted to partner with had a Ph.D. in raw vegan nutritional healing, which dovetailed nicely with his Reiki certification. He pitched it to me by saying that, since I would not let him live out his dream by moving, he needed something to engage in. Something about it didn't feel quite right, but I figured that it was better than having him unemployed.

Myra

Pat spoke a lot about how our greatest goal in life should be to love and help others. He spoke about God and forgiveness, and how we had to forgive other people in order to be free. He went on to further explain how God puts people in our lives who we can help if we so choose. I wholeheartedly agreed with these principles, but something felt off to me. I felt like he was manipulating me somehow which, of course, he was.

Myra, a single mother with two children—who was in a financial crisis—was the woman Pat wanted to start a business with. According to him, she needed to save up money so they could start their business. I agreed to meet the woman, and when I pressed Pat further to tell me who she really was—because I had a feeling she was his ex—I learned that yes, Myra was the woman he had cheated on me with, and who he had dated for a few months after I kicked him out. Pat convinced me that he had never really felt anything more than friendship for her and there was nothing between them. He also said that going into business with her was his only option because he could not afford to do it alone.

Most people would think I was completely out of my mind, and maybe I was, but I chose to look at Myra as a human being and not as my boyfriend's ex. She and I talked, and she apologized for what happened. She said Pat had told her that he and I were already broken up when they started dating, and that there was nothing between them anymore. She told me of how he'd always spoken of me while they were together, and that she felt he'd never stopped loving me. She was actually quite a lovely, educated person, and she offered to help me with nutritional counseling to help with my health.

I felt torn. I wanted to be the person who takes the high road, forgives, lets things go, and doesn't hold onto grudges. That seemed like an evolved way of being, and I felt helping another human being was the right thing to do. Besides, it was too much work to argue because my head hurt too much, and the fog in my head was unrelenting. In my heart, I had forgiven Pat for cheating—and I forgave Myra for her part in it—but my heart was still hurt and scarred. Pat told me that forgiving means completely erasing what has been done, but although I was no longer angry with him, I couldn't quite buy that forgiving meant completely *forgetting*. Nevertheless, I let it go. I also agreed to let Myra and her two kids move into our basement for six months. Myra had a new boyfriend who would be joining them which made things easier to accept, as Myra and her boyfriend seemed quite happy together.

They moved in roughly two and a half months after my accident. I was functioning a little better by then, but I still could not work nor do much around the house because fatigue engulfed my very pores. I would go places, like for a walk or to a store, and not remember what I was doing there, how I had gotten there, or even where I was. Cooking a meal was overwhelming because it would suck the energy out of me and I kept forgetting what I was doing. I had a nasty habit of leaving the stove on and walking away, and more than a few things got burnt. Eventually, I had to step away from the stove for a while.

Myra stepped right in and helped with everything, which was a relief to me. Pat had even started helping out more. Any doubts I had about the two of them were washed away, mostly because I didn't have the energy to think about it.

Within a month, Pat started acting strange again. He decided to leave to drive up north for a few days right when I had to have another surgery on my foot. For some strange reason, one of the larger lateral screws from the metal plate had migrated over to the adjacent bone, and the screws that were on top had started popping out. It was painful, and made it hard to walk. They had to redo the entire fusion, and I was back in a cast again. The surgeon told me she had never seen anything like it.

By now, I was frustrated with having so many surgeries, and I was tired of hearing doctors tell me how unusual my symptoms were—but as always, my relationship drama took precedence. I began to have this feeling that Pat still had feelings for Myra, because he was acting more odd than usual, so, I confronted him. Because of the brain fog, I don't remember exactly how everything unfolded—but I discovered that Pat had actually recently proposed to Myra, and that she had said yes. He'd convinced her that he no longer loved me, and had wooed her until she broke up with her boyfriend. Then they had agreed not to act on their feelings until they had moved out together, to spare my feelings. So the man I had let back into my life, and stranger I opened my home to, had both put knives in my back.

It felt as if the whole world was crashing down around me. The fog in my head was thicker than ever, and I felt like a corpse. I was confused and could not grasp what was happening, or how it had even started. Once again that dark presence enveloped my soul. I wanted out of this life. I didn't want this pain anymore. I did not want to be hurt by people anymore. I didn't want any more illnesses or injuries or surgeries. I had enough of all the men who'd hurt me. I couldn't stand being betrayed, lied to and played for a fool anymore. I hated the fact that I was so gullible and naïve, and had such a hard time saying no to people, who then took advantage of me. Why were things so hard and so unfair? I prayed for death. I begged for death. I planned for death. I felt utterly hopeless, and that there truly was no hope of me ever finding real love.

I remember confronting Myra and Pat. At that moment, some of the pea soup fog in my brain cleared enough for me to see just how mentally ill Pat was. I had failed to see it in its wholeness before. Myra did not know that Pat had proposed to me only four months before that. He said he was in love with both of us and didn't want to have to choose between us, so he left. In his insane narcissism, it's conceivable he had actually planned all along to have the two women he supposedly loved under one roof, in the hope that we would share him. I was angry, hurt, devastated, disgusted, and horrified all at the same time. Myra was livid and said she never wanted to have anything to do with him again.

I went to my room and sat on the floor, paralyzed and unable to move. Then the tears came. I didn't think I had any left as it seemed like my entire relationship with Pat had dried up every ounce. I sat heaving heavy sobs for hours on the floor, unable to move. Here I was, the star in my very own psychological horror movie. I was in so much shock, not so much about what had happened, but more about how I'd ended up being broken, hurt and confused beyond belief. It felt like I was in some kind of soap opera—and I was the director. Had I really let myself sink this low for love? Was I that desperate? Had I *really* been so blind and naive? The answer was yes, yes, and yes.

A hollow self-loathing whirled inside me like a tornado, stirring up every emotion imaginable for days afterward. My children were with their father that week, and so I shut myself off from the world. I could not pretend, or hide my feelings, from anyone at that point. I could not even look at myself in the mirror. I was filled with disgust; Pat was gone, but I was stuck with Myra and her two kids in my house. In some ways, the betrayal from her hurt a lot more than the betrayal from Pat. I was used to feeling belittled and rejected by him, but Myra had seemed like a friend.

I told her she had to move out, but that I would give her a month because of the children. She agreed but insisted that we talk.

In the arms of the darkness, I concocted an elaborate foolproof plan to end my life, and then wound up flipflopping back and forth between putting myself out of my misery and facing the situation. I went so far as to drive up north one night with a bottle of wine, charcoal, and a small fire pit. I was going to build a nice charcoal fire in my car and drink enough to fall asleep never wake up as the so that the carbon monoxide ended my life peacefully. In a dark parking lot behind an old country church, I drank the wine to give me the nerve to go through with it. Those old, familiar whispers trying to convince me that there I would finally be at peace, with no more suffering or pain, were enticing. All I had to do was light that match. But something inside of me rebelled. No! I didn't really want to die; I just wanted my suffering to end. I did not want to have to be strong anymore in a world of heartless people.

But how could I move forward? I didn't want to fight my battles alone anymore; it was just too hard. Hours went by as I argued in my head until, between the wine and the brain fog, I fell asleep.

When I awoke early the next morning, the push to end my life had dissipated. Arriving home, I agreed to talk to Myra. The conversation lasted for hours, and then continued into the ensuing weeks. We were so much alike it was scary. We were both deeply broken inside, desperate to feel love, had no personal boundaries, and had utterly low feelings of self-worth that we masked by being outwardly happy and appearing well put-together. Pat's charm, romance, lies, and manipulation had put a spell on each of us; we had both fallen in love with a narcissistic manipulative abuser who had bipolar disorder.

Eventually, I would go on to read books about abusers and victims, and it was quite a shock to realize that I was a textbook victim. Pat was the most charming, romantic man I had ever met when we first started dating. He had a magnetic quality to him that was like a drug I became addicted to. Then he started taking it away, bit by bit, until the charm and romance only came out when he knew I was withdrawing from him. Throughout the relationship, Pat had managed to convince me that things were my fault, and that if I'd only behave a certain way, he wouldn't need to get so angry. This fostered feelings of guilt and increasing self-doubt in me, which evolved into self-loathing and the feeling that I needed him more than water. It happened so slowly, and he was so methodical in his manipulation, that I didn't even realize it until the rug was pulled out from under my feet and I was lying on the floor.

Everything, including all his verbal abuse, was an attempt to manipulate and control me. I became isolated from my friends and family because he would act hurt or jealous when I saw them. Later on in the relationship, I was simply too embarrassed to bring him anywhere in case he had a manic outburst. No wonder he'd wanted me to move with him far away from the city; he wanted me isolated from everyone I knew so he could continue to assert dominance over me. No one in my life, up until that point, knew what was going on—although I think some suspected it. Strangely, it was actually a huge relief to talk to Myra about it. However, she had only experienced his abuse over the few months they were together, while for me it had been over four years of my life; four years that my self-esteem had been buried in the ground until there were no more tears left to cry; four years that I would never get back.

For the time being, I pushed aside what Myra had done because I knew she was just as much, or even more, broken than I was. But as naive and gullible as we both were to fall for Pat—and in my case to stay with him for so long—I would *never* have been so blinded by my own neediness to stuck a knife in someone's back like she did to me. I befriended her and let her family stay with me so they could get back on their feet, and I was betrayed.

However, despite everything, Myra and I needed each other for that season in our lives. Stress and brain injuries don't go well together and my brain was so messed up, scattered, and forgetful that, while I needed to talk to someone about my feelings, there was no way I could even *think* about speaking to anyone else but her, not even a therapist. I was too overwhelmed with humiliation and shame, and too physically broken as well.

The time between Pat moving out and Myra moving out was a time of self-exploration and healing for both of us, and we helped each other through it as we unpacked all the details of our respective relationships with Pat. We laughed. We cried. We lamented. I knew there was no way I could ever stay friends with her afterward, but we served a purpose for each other during that time. Like me, she was filled with shame and regret. Sometimes we would just sit on the couch, absolutely dumbfounded about the whole situation. It didn't seem real.

I'm so thankful that my children never knew what had happened with Pat. I was so ashamed of myself, and so was Myra. How could we even begin to tell anybody what had happened? We just couldn't.

God

Myra moved out. We remained in sporadic contact, until it eventually flickered out. She would go on to jump into other toxic relationships, and eventually move out of the country. As for me, I was determined to remain single. I had jumped from one toxic relationship to the next for my entire adult life, and enough was enough! Time and time again I had gone against my intuition; in fact, in almost every relationship I had ever been in, I'd ignored the little voice inside me that told me it was wrong. I knew I had work to do, and I could not repeat the same patterns.

Some people might say it was bad luck that I ended up with all the wrong men, but I know it went much deeper than that. Even though I didn't deserve to be treated the way I'd been treated, I'd allowed it to happen. I couldn't blame anyone else for the choices I had made.

Friends continually told me how much I inspired them because I was so strong and had overcome so much. They remarked on how I always seemed peaceful, happy and compassionate. Inside, I laughed a sarcastic snicker at this because outwardly, I suppose I appeared positive, but I had learned from a young age to just 'get on with it' as the expression goes, and I was good at masking my feelings and thoughts.

People ask me how I stayed so positive with so much trouble in my life, and I sometimes think that perhaps, somewhere in the depths of my soul, I knew things would be okay and that is what kept pushing me forward. Still, at the time I split with Pat—and Myra—I could not tell anyone the truth of what had transpired during that relationship, and where it had left me. I just couldn't.

Telling people the truth would have destroyed the image that I had worked so hard on presenting to the world. I liked that people saw me as being strong but kind, resilient and able to triumph through adversity, but the truth was that mostly I was a broken, lost soul full of self-doubt, fear, and insecurity. I feared that if people saw the true me, they would see a crazy woman and run. I realized that I had let the state of every relationship I'd ever been in dictate my state of mind, to the point that my identity and feelings of self-worth were determined by how well things were going. I was a hypocrite who would never allow my friends to be treated badly, yet I had become my own worst enemy.

As I reflected, I realized that one of the things that kept me going back to Pat was his pursuit of spirituality. All of his talk about higher powers sparked something deep inside of me, even though something didn't feel quite right about him from the onset. I needed to know the truth about God. Where was He in all of this, and how did He fit into my life? This yearning got deeper and deeper.

I didn't know where to get answers, so I started to read the Bible. Years prior, I had attempted to read it, but it had been a King James version, which I found it too hard for my injured brain to read and comprehend. Because I had a sense that I was being prompted to read it, this time, I found an easy-to-read version. I also started searching for bipolar and abuse support groups. Perhaps speaking with other victims of abuse would help me.

My internet search led me to a site in another country, which had a link to a church not too far from me. I called the church to get more information and was connected with the pastor. He told me he had been planning to start a support group, but in the midst of it had been called to move away. I told him a little bit about my relationship with Pat, which was very hard for me to do. His voice was filled with compassion, and he asked if he could pray with me over the phone. I agreed, and he asked God to help me through the situation and for God to work in my heart so that I would come to know how truly loved I was.

No one had ever prayed out loud just for me. Those words washed over me like a tidal wave and left me in tears. But they were not tears of sadness, they were tears of realization that maybe, just maybe there was hope. As he continued to pray, I felt an overwhelming sense of peace and a yearning inside of me for more. But I worried, how could God love me after all I had done? Besides, I was hardly a Christian. Growing up, I had gone to a Catholic school and sometimes with my family to mass at Christmas, Easter, or school functions—but that was the extent of my experience. I knew nothing of other Christian faiths. He told me a little bit about his church and invited me to come. It would be another two months before I would go.

In the meantime, I had another pressing matter. It has been almost eight months since the accident and I was still not ready to go back to work full time. I had tried, and was currently working four hours a day, twice a week—and even this seemed like a lot for my brain to handle.

On workdays, I would end up exhausted, in a dark room, unable to do anything for the rest of the day. It scared me. I had moments of clarity where I could see how messed up I really was, and I also had moments of guilt at not being able to be the kind of mother my children needed. Instead of playing games, reading, or watching movies with them, I sank lower into my mattress. They had already been through so many ups, downs and surgeries with me, that it didn't seem fair that their mother was now reduced to being a total 'couch potato'.

I tried to act normal and do family things, and sometimes that worked in short spurts, but it always came with the hefty price tag of a blinding headache, nausea, brain fog, dizziness, and fatigue. Still, I could not, and *would* not give in. At work, I slowly worked myself up from two days a week to four, but it was still *so* challenging. I could function for a little while, but then fatigue and headaches set in, and the fog in my brain became as thick as pea soup.

On the very limited income I had from my auto insurance claim, I could no longer afford my house in the city. My disability insurer cut off my benefits four weeks after the car accident, and so I had to hire a lawyer. My car had been hit at 100 kilometers per hour while I was at a stop; between the heavy impact, the fact that my car was a write-off, my pre-existing medical history, and the injuries I sustained in the accident, it was utterly bewildering that they could cut me off without even seeing me. But they did. Even the doctor I was seeing at the brain injury clinic was appalled. It was yet another battle I had to fight that I had no energy for.

There was no choice, I had to sell my house and find something cheaper. The only way to do that was to move out of the city. I would have to leave my friends and family and everything familiar. My children were devastated, and I felt horrible. They had already been through so much with me, either waiting for a surgery or recovering from one—but when I looked at the pile of bills, I could see no other alternative. My real estate agent was absolutely fantastic, and so compassionate. We saw over 100 houses. I could only handle seeing four or five at a time and would sleep in his car on the way back, because my brain would just get overwhelmed and shut off.

During the time of the house hunt, I finally decided to go to that new church. I remember walking in the door and immediately feeling that this was undoubtedly the place I needed to be. It was unlike anything I had ever experienced before. It was lively, the music was amazing, and it felt like home despite there being a ton of people. Surrounded by my new church friends, I began praying every day, asking God to lead me to the house where *He* wanted me to be, and not where *I* wanted to be. Instead of me controlling my life, I handed over the reins to God, and I felt complete trust in Him. Doing things my way hadn't worked out so well and I figured that if he made me, he knew what was best for me.

One day my real estate agent and I were on our way to put in an offer on a house, but he wanted to show me one more that had just come onto the market. It was a little back split in a very quiet residential neighborhood, and much farther away from the city than I had hoped, so I was felt a little unsure about it. Before we even stepped in the door, I had a feeling it was the one I was meant to have, although I did not *want* it to be the one. The price was very good, because everything inside it screamed the 1970s, including wood paneling in the basement, shag carpet, and green walls. In my head I asked, "Really God, *this*?"

Even though I knew this was the house I was supposed to get, I asked God for a sign to prove it. No sooner than I had uttered the prayer, when the owner's dog came running out of a room to greet me—and it was a carbon copy of my own little dog. I walked around the house, thinking it was too big for just me and my girls and that I really didn't want another fixer upper, and then I asked God for another sign. We left the house, drove around the neighborhood and wouldn't you know it, one street over was a street named after me: Susan Crescent. We put in the offer that night, and the next day it was accepted.

My city house sold within three days for well over the asking price, and my financial worries were over. I cried as I signed the papers because, even though I knew I *had* to leave, I did not want to leave my neighborhood. All my friends were so close by, and so were my parents. Moving would mean starting over alone, with no friends or family close by. It was scary, ultimately I placed my trust in God, knowing that he would somehow use it for good.

We moved into our new home in August. I was not ready to get to know the neighbours, and so I barely went out or spoke to anyone. I felt I needed time on my own to figure out exactly who I was, and why my life had turned out the way it had. I read my Bible, I started seeing a therapist, and I spoke to pastors. I gave my life to Jesus and got baptized. I came to understand that Jesus saw into my soul, saw all the mistakes I had made, and met me with overwhelming love, grace, and forgiveness. He forgave me for trying to take my own life. He forgave me for cheating, and for all the casual sex. He forgave me for living a lie, and all the masks I wore. He forgave me for turning away from Him. He loved me so much that He gave his life for me, a sinner who did not deserve it. I wanted to become more like Him. I knew that to do that, I had to forgive everyone who had ever hurt me … and I had to forgive myself for those I had hurt. It took a long time, but I did, and the sense of peace and freedom I felt was a new, wonderful experience.

By September I was hosting a weekly 'connect group' that consisted of eleven other members of our church and me. We could come together to study and share life, and after a few weeks, I told the group about my head injury and my daily struggles with headaches, fatigue, and brain fog. They offered to pray over me, and all eleven members put their hands on either my head, shoulder, or arm and took turns praying. I felt a little strange because suddenly I had all this attention and I'd never experienced anything remotely close to this before. Then suddenly, in the middle of it, I saw a flash of white light—and just like that, my symptoms were suddenly gone! I still had my physical pain but the brain fog that had been consuming me for 14 months had dissipated, and the headaches were gone. I could function!

Up until that moment, I was still only working four hours a day and struggling cognitively but happiness was something I could now see in my future. I went back to work full time the following week, and three years later I am still working full time. I still get fatigued or have the occasional headache when I am overwhelmed, and my memory is not the greatest, especially when I am tired or over-stimulated; however, the difference is like night and day!

I was so grateful to be able to function, but I was curious and a little upset that, if God could miraculously heal my brain, why couldn't he heal the rest of me just as miraculously? Why only a little, and not all the way? Why did he not make the chronic pain go away? It is human nature to always want more than what we are given.

I had this feeling in me that there was a purpose to my struggles. I knew God could heal me, but there was a bigger picture that maybe one day I would see, so I trusted in that. He would give me the strength I needed to keep going.

We live in a world that is beyond broken, and full of bad things, but God gave us free will and the ability to make choices. People have both good and bad in them, and one small choice can tip the scales to set a chain of events into motion that can be good or bad depending on the choice. If one person makes a bad choice, it can yield ripples into the future that we may not even be able to see. Such choices are often made because humanity has become very self-focused. We live in an age of 'what's in it for me?', and many of us distract ourselves in social media, or binge-watching shows, so we don't have to think about the choices we have made, or the consequences.

When something bad happens, there are endless questions. For example, when a loved one dies people ask, "How could God let my loved one suffer? How could He allow the violence or disease that took my loved one?" I don't have the answers, but I am sure of one thing; God does not choose to let us suffer. We set that up ourselves.

Parents try to teach their children right from wrong, and do their best to protect them. They tell them not to put dirt in their mouths, or to stop running because the floor is wet and they will fall, but they do it anyway. We pick them up, wipe their tears and tell them we love them, all the while knowing that when they reach adulthood, they will live their lives the way they think is best, no matter what we taught them.

So it is with God and us, His children. He gave us life and this world. He taught us right from wrong. But we choose to do what we think is best, we think we know better than the one who created us. He still loves us even when, like me, we run on the wet floors and fall. I was that child, and I did not know that God was always there to wipe away my tears and hold me. I could not feel Him, because I could not stop myself long enough to listen. I was too busy distracting myself, and following my own will, even when I knew without a doubt that this was not the life God had planned for me.

My mother spent many years angry with God, asking Him why He took my brother away. I understand that, like all of us, my brother had choices. Some bad things happened in his life, often because of other broken people; maybe in his own pain he sometimes hurt other people. Maybe this accumulation of things, added to his Chron's disease, tipped the scale, which resulted in him ending his life. Maybe the chemistry in his brain was off, and it was just his time. I don't know the answers, but I do know that God is not to blame.

I could easily look at my own life and ask God why I have had so many health problems, and why he let me go through so much trauma with the wrong kind of men … but I already know the answer. If we lived in a perfect world, nothing bad would ever happen, but in a perfect world, there would have to be perfect people, and the only perfect person to ever walk the Earth was brutally murdered, tortured and nailed to a cross. So 'imperfect me' made some not so perfect choices, adding to my existing brokenness. Does that explain my health conditions? Not really, but it gives me peace about the fact that bad stuff just happens. It also helps me to understand that God is there alongside us on the paths we walk, and that good can come out of even the worst tragedies. God does not cause bad things to happen. They just happen.

Through my deepening commitment to a Christian walk, an inward journey began. I started looking at everything that had happened in my life through a different lens. I realized that, when I was told that I would never walk again, I'd learned to be perseverant and resilient, and more importantly, how to be a fighter. Recovering from surgeries in bed taught me patience and self-care. The challenges of having mild ADHD forced me to learn to sit still. Witnessing a screaming man in a store triggered compassion in me, I knew what mental illness felt like. And my brother's suicide allowed me to be there with understanding and compassion for someone who experienced something similar.

The abusive relationship with Pat, as much as it drained me, ultimately led me to finding not only myself, but God. It resulted in me finally seeing myself as worthy through the eyes of my creator. Would I be where I am today if it weren't for all of these things that transpired? It's impossible to know, because I have not yet reached the end of my journey; there is still so much in store for me.

I did not date, or even think about dating, for almost a year and a half after Pat left for good. This was a record for me. Pat emailed me a few times, trying to get back together, but I saw him with different eyes now. He said he too had become a Christian, and that God had changed him. He had even moved into my city for a few months, I guess in hopes of reconnecting. I met with him a couple of times, but only because I needed to truly know that I had forgiven him. I wanted closure on those chapters of my life.

When I met with Pat, it was painful. I learned that—although he had indeed changed—he was still mentally ill, he refused to seek medical attention for his disease, and he was still a narcissist. Just as when we were together, he seemed to feel it was his mission to help people see the error of their ways. The difference now was that I felt a new strength in me and realized that he no longer had a hold on me. Even if he had been on medication and was stable, there was no way I would have gone back; the scars in my heart were just too deep. I knew God had different plans for me.

The meetings I had with him allowed me to see the extent of his disease. He was able to share a bit about his illness and told me how he could create a version of reality for himself that became so real to him that he could not differentiate between truth and fantasy. He had hidden it from me for the first year of our relationship to lure me in. I let go of the guilt I felt for having gotten involved with him in the first place. He had a serious mental illness. During our time together, my inflated ego had actually believed I could fix him, but now I cared about myself and knew I would never allow myself to be treated badly again. I also felt compassion for him, because I truly believed he was not capable of love while we were together.

Seeing him also brought back memories of his abuse; he hacked into my computer several times and monitored me, even when we were apart and he destroyed precious photographs and personal documents in his jealous rage. The worst thing he did, the one thing that hit me the hardest, was to throw out a journal I'd made with all the funny, cute things my children had said or done throughout their loves. He'd just thrown it away without telling me. Because of my memory problems, most of those stories still have not come back to me.

Pat made some attempts to try to lure me in again, but I was different now. I told him once and for all that although I had forgiven him, I could never be in his life again. I felt proud for standing firm and respecting myself. I could have blamed him for everything that had happened, but at the end of the day, I was the one who kept taking him back. I had to take responsibility too.

Pat seemed to respect my decision, although he looked hurt. A couple of months went by and I heard nothing from him, and I was glad and relieved to think that he was out of my life completely ... until one day his ex-wife got in contact with me, and I had a long, eye-opening conversation with her that made me grateful God had removed Pat from my life, even though I kept taking him back. From her, I learned the extent of his lies—which pretty much extended into every aspect of the relationship we had, and everything he'd ever told me. She told me he had beaten her many times, and even put her in the hospital a few times. He had even hit his kids—and that was when she left him.

It was shocking to hear these things, and I felt betrayed and foolish all over again. During the course of our relationship, I'd questioned many times whether he'd been bipolar all along, or if his behavior was a result of the accident. His ex-wife answered that question. Though he'd convinced me his bipolar condition was triggered by his injury—and I chose to believe it—it was not the car accident after all. He was very sick.

Feelings of shame tried to creep inside my head, but by now I knew how to dispel that voice by praying. I wasn't the only woman who was deceived. Pat had deceived his ex-wife too, and she was an educated woman. I thanked God that I didn't share any children with him, and that he had never hurt mine. His own children had suffered greatly, but his ex-wife told me they had been in counseling and were doing well.

Quite out of the blue, a few months later Pat showed up at my door in tears apologizing for everything he had done. I had already forgiven him, but it was nice to hear, and he seemed sincere. But his very next sentence was, "I forgive you too." *What?* This came as a complete shock. *Forgive me for what?* I had been a silent doormat who had been supportive, doting and loving all through our relationship while he had taken complete advantage of me.

I took a step back and realized that this was just another attempt to manipulate me. I didn't even bother asking what it was I had supposedly done that required his forgiveness, because I knew in my heart I had done nothing wrong to him. In fact, the person I had wronged was *myself*! I told him politely that I never wanted to see or hear from him again, and he left saying that he would always love me and be there for me if I ever changed my mind. He told me that in his heart, I would always be his wife. I turned away and locked my door. I never heard from him again.

For almost the next two years, I remained single and it was one of the best times of my life. I went out occasionally with friends from church, but other than that I spent most of my time alone. I attended talk therapy, and did a lot of soul-searching which, though it was hard to admit, showed me clearly that I had been jumping from one codependent relationship to the next. I'd read about codependency in my psychology books, but I had never seen myself that way—yet there it was: In all my relationships, I'd been excessively reliant on my partners for approval and my sense of identity. Through my desperate need to feel loved, I'd lost my sense of self. I'd tried to mold myself into the person I thought my partners wanted me to be, enabling them to take advantage of me.

As I unpacked these pieces of myself, I realized that my self-worth had been so completely wrapped up in how other people saw me that I gravitated toward men who were not capable of loving me back. How had I let myself be treated so badly? How had I sunk so low?

My therapist had mentioned that it seemed that, right from childhood, I'd had a fundamental belief that I was not lovable and, as a result, I instinctively gravitated toward people who fostered that belief. I'd heard this several times, but it had not really sunk in before. It was hard to digest … yet I knew it to be true. I had subconsciously chosen men who could not love me, yet I wanted so badly to feel loved. The beauty of my Christian faith was that, when I realized God's love was more than enough, I stopped looking for a man to fill the void in my heart and came to understand that, no matter how perfect a partner I found, he would never be able to complete me.

This new knowledge completely contradicted my lifetime fantasy of 'happily ever after', a deeply ingrained notion I'd gotten from years of reading romance novels and watching 'happily ever after' movies. I finally let go of the idea that by finding a perfect partner, I would be complete. Instead, I accepted that life is a roller coaster full of ups and downs; became grateful for the joy of happy moments, and the lessons from bad moments; and, accepted that I was already complete.

Something else happened during my solitude period that greatly changed my life. I hesitate to write this because I know most people won't believe it. I went through something called 'restoration prayer' (some call it deliverance) at my church. It is akin to what's generally known as an exorcism … and it literally changed my life.

All my life, I had voices whispering in my ear, telling me that I was not good enough, not lovable, and that I should just end my life. My entire life, it felt like something was trying to control me. I can remember these voices as early as when I was seven years old, sitting on the rooftop of our house, pondering jumping. It would come on suddenly. I would feel fine one minute, and then suddenly I would make a mistake—like burn dinner—and the voices would come flooding in, telling me I was worthless and couldn't do anything right, and that I should end my life. But then the feeling would disappear, and I'd be normal … until the next time. After the restoration prayer, these voices were completely gone.

Some might call it negative energy, but I firmly believe that up until that point of my life, I was surrounded and infected by demons. After the restoration prayer, it literally felt like black tar had been removed from my insides. The dark stain that had seemed to be fighting for my soul was gone. All thoughts about wanting to end my life, even in my lowest moments, never returned. All of the dark thoughts about my unworthiness were completely gone, never to return.

Of course during this process I could not help but think of the conversation I'd had with my father about how he'd summoned a demon to get my mother to marry him, and after my own healing from the darkness, I knew beyond a shadow of a doubt that the devil was *real*. There were too many unexplained things in my life for me not to believe it; all the dark, moving shapes I sometimes saw, or the sense that my mind was playing tricks on me finally made sense.

I'm not blaming every bad thing that happened in my life on this darkness, but I do believe it played a part. Despite the darkness whispering in my ear, I was the one who made the poor choices, and I was responsible for those choices. Now, however, with the demons and their whispers gone, I could finally move forward with my life. The surreal feeling of freedom I felt transcends words.

God saved me. God loves me. He loved me all along, and always will. Through my faith, I came to see myself as He sees me, and that changed me and put me on a new path. Yes, therapy helped me deal with mental and physical issues … but it was my *soul* that needed tending to. Through my Christian faith, I learned without a doubt that God doesn't make mistakes … which means that I am not a mistake, a mistaken belief I had in my heart that held me back. God forgave me for the sins of my past … but now I had to forgive myself, not only for hurting others, but for hurting myself. But I realized that, if God loved me so much that He could forgive me, then I must.

As part of my healing journey, I would go on long meditation walks. Often, I would be so enamored with the beauty around me that just looking at a tree would bring tears of joy, awe, and wonderment. Many believe in a higher power, but looking at nature confirms it for me. To be surrounded by such beauty, there *has* to have been a conscious creator, just the same way that a paint has to have a painter. It is impossible to come from nothing. It is unfathomable that everything appeared by accident. As I came to embrace the idea that God created me for a reason, inner peace and contentment filled me. I was still riding a roller coaster of emotions, but inside me I knew I would be okay, and that I would never reach those self-destructive lows again. And I have not, to this very day.

I kept working at growing my walk with God, and more and more positive realizations kept coming at me. I was changing—but it was really God who was working in me, because every day I would pray, "Lord, make me into the woman you created me to be." That is still my daily prayer.

It was not instant change. I had sad moments when I would curl up in a ball on the sofa in the living room and just cry, because part of me still wanted to feel sorry for all that had happened to me. But I only allowed myself to cry for a little bit; I would not linger in it. It is okay to allow ourselves to shed a few tears now and then. When the crying was done, I knew it was time to focus on the solution, and put what I'd learned to use!

I read a book on boundaries, and it was quite an eye-opener for me. I came to understand that I'd never had any boundaries and that my inability to say no had gotten me into far too much trouble. In fact, I realized that many of my relationships had started only because I could not say 'no' to the men who pursued me—even when I didn't really want to be with them. My 'modus operandi' had been to just go along with things because I was afraid to let people down in case they wouldn't like me anymore. It seems odd to me now that I would want a person to like me, even though I wanted to break up with them!

In retrospect, it's clear that I felt afraid to establish boundaries because it was so foreign to me. Would people still like me if I didn't agree with them? That inability to say no to people started in childhood, and even today it is still a part of me. However, now I understand it and know how to deal with it. I started small. If someone would ask something of me, or invite me to go somewhere and I couldn't do it or didn't want to, I would very gently say, "No, thank you," without trying to justify myself or my decision. It was gratifying to learn that no one got upset with me for saying 'no'! However, while it became easier to establish healthy boundaries with friends and family, the real test would come when I started dating.

After a year-and-a-half, I felt ready to do just that. While I was content being single, and prepared to remain that way, in my heart I wanted a husband to share my life with. I wasn't lonely but I thought it would be nice to find someone, and so I made a list of all the qualities I wanted my future husband to have. Then I told myself, *if I don't find someone who checks off all the boxes, I will remain single,* and I prayed to God to give me strength.

Alberto

I put an ad on a local dating site. It was lengthy and very straightforward in terms of what I was searching for in a partner, and what I could offer. At the end of my ad, I added a question for respondents to answer; it was a test to see if people had actually read my full profile, and to find out if they were interested in knowing *me* as opposed to simply looking at my picture to see if they found me attractive. The ones who responded with a simple, "Hi, how are you?" had clearly not read my profile, and so I just deleted their messages.

As a Christian, and a grateful one at that, one key criteria for the man I wanted was that he had to share my faith. I love going to church alone or with friends, but I felt strongly that if I was to be in a relationship, I wanted my man to be sitting beside me, and praying with me. If I could not find that, then I was happy to be alone.

One hears many stories of dating horrors—and I certainly have my own—but this time God was with me and surprisingly, I mostly had good experiences. As I searched for a partner who I would be well matched with, I met several different men. We would chat for a bit on the internet and then meet up for a coffee date. When I was not interested in someone, it was difficult for me to get the words out to say so because, in my subconscious, I secretly still wanted people to like me, and it pained me to think they were mad at me. But I did it. And it did upset one man. I went on two dates with him and knew he was not for me, but when I told him, he was hurt said angrily that there was just no one decent out there, and that he was going to give up dating. By now I could smell codependency and it sickened me. I blocked his number.

There was another man who I had spent a long time talking on the phone with. We had a lot in common, our conversations were great, and it seemed like we shared the same faith and the values. And then we met. He was forty pounds heavier than the five-year-old picture of himself that he had posted, not to mention four inches shorter than he claimed to be. I was disappointed—not because he was short and heavy, but because he had lied to me. I began to doubt whether I should be dating at all.

I began getting quite ruthless about who I would date. For example, I couldn't stand pictures of middle-aged men, standing shirtless in front of a bathroom mirror, who said they were 'looking for a long-term relationship'. I just skipped through those. I also was ruthless about my new moral code. Most people want to have sex after a few dates, but I was determined to wait for marriage. I wanted to be friends first and really get to know someone before taking the step into intimacy. I'd learned from my past experiences that jumping into bed too quickly established a level of intimacy that set the tone for the relationship that followed, with a focus physicality instead of real intimacy. I couldn't do that anymore.

Some men were shocked to hear this from me, and turned me away. Some tried to change my mind. Some were absolutely thrilled and thought I was another Mother Theresa, just because I decided to respect my body and hold true to my values—sorry, I am not a saint.

I got disillusioned after a while because I was not able to find what I was looking for. After a few more weeks of trying, dating started to become a chore. I still hadn't found what I was looking for, so I suspended my profile. There was no way that I would ever 'settle' again.

Shortly after that, there came an evening when I stood in my backyard, by my overgrown vegetable garden, with my list in hand. I held it up to the sky and thanked God for everything He had given me. I told him I was happy, but that I wanted a husband who met my list of requirements, or I would have no husband at all. The next day I had the urge to check my messages one last time and there was a message from Alberto. After a few text messages and phone conversations, we agreed to meet.

Alberto was very different from the men I had been with before. He was very easy to talk to, and our coffee turned to dinner. In the weeks that followed, we spent spend hours upon hours chatting on the phone, if we weren't together. He was smart, handsome, had a good job, was not embroiled in any ugly custody battles, was part of a good circle of family and friends, called himself a Christian, was honest and trustworthy, and tolerated my corny sense of humor. He also knew about my chronic pain and the fact that my ankylosing spondylitis was an incurable and progressive disease. This did not deter him. He said he was into health and nutrition, as I was. It felt right. He checked off the boxes on my lengthy list, and so three weeks later—when he asked me to marry him—I said, "Yes."

It felt a little crazy, but *right*. I even asked God for signs that this was His will and not my own, and He gave them to me. The apartment building Alberto lived in turned out to be the same building I had lived in with Juan when I was pregnant with our first daughter. Not only that, but he lived on the same floor, in very next unit. A street in my neighborhood was named after his daughter, Sophia. Juan's best friend had dated Alberto's ex-wife many years prior, so they all knew each other. To me, that seemed like confirmation.

Alberto's ex-wife, who was also a Christian, was a wonderful woman. We became fast friends. Also, all of my friends and family liked Alberto. However, the single most important factor for me in agreeing to marry him was that he agreed that praying and going to church together was important to him, and the kind of life he wanted. Everything just felt like it fell into place.

Of course, everyone was a little shocked to find out I got engaged after only three weeks; still, after all I had been through, and all the work I had done to heal myself, I felt this was the path God wanted me to take.

Alberto and I went for premarital counseling at my church. The pastor, who was also a psychologist, said that we would end up triggering each other, but that if we can recognize our triggers, as well as our responses to those triggers, God uses our spouses to help us grow. How right he was; I am triggered by anger and blame. It ignites old, ingrained feelings in me of not being lovable. When I am triggered I withdraw emotionally, or get defensive. In turn, when I withdraw it triggers Alberto's feelings of abandonment—and he reacts with anger and withdrawal. Not a fun dance, and to this day we struggle.

We both felt we were capable of handling *any* situation because we were in love. What we did not realize was that we would end up triggering the heck out of each other—and that, while recognizing triggers and responses is a good first step, putting healthy, productive behaviors into action in the heat of an argument is extremely challenging. However, we both try.

The next step was blending our families. We both had shared custody arrangements with our former spouses. My daughters were eleven and sixteen. His children were three, twelve, and fourteen. When we introduced them, the first few meetings were somewhat awkward, as expected, but in a short time, we all became very close. I knew everything would be fine.

The wedding took place in my church. I wanted a private destination wedding without a lot of fuss, but Alberto wanted something a little bigger. Ultimately, his family flew in from

Mexico and we had about 50 friends and family attend the ceremony and reception afterward.

Everything went smoothly. We had a romantic honeymoon and then Alberto moved into my house. It was an adjustment, to say the least. We had only known each other for six months by the time we got married, and while he was a kind and decent man, we were opposite in so many things. He liked the bed made perfectly; I never made mine. He liked to take time to think about things, especially when we would argue; I liked to settle things before we went to sleep. He was highly logical and analytical; I was a bit impulsive and made decisions primarily based on emotions. He was a strict parent; I was not. He had said he was into exercise and healthy eating (as I was my whole life), but in fact, he was not; he overate and did not exercise, and by the time we got married, he'd put on an extra 25 pounds.

The things I respect most about Alberto are how he strives for continuous self-improvement, how perseverant he is, and how important family is to him. Like me, he has his flaws and I have to fight an impulse to want to 'fix' them. Luckily, I am able to quickly recognize old destructive behavior patterns and send them away. I do my best not to have any expectations, because expectations lead to disappointment. This is what many books I've read tell me. They also say that love is unconditional, not necessarily reciprocal, and selfless.

I thought I had that part nailed, but it turns out that it's more difficult than I thought. I mean, we all have some type of expectation; for example, I expect my husband to be faithful and honest. But what is the scope of honesty? If he is not honest with me about some things, do I still love him?

The Bible tells me what love is in 1 Corinthians 13. It's all nicely laid out there, and boy do I want to love that way ... but my wicked human heart seems to want to go against this at times. I am still grappling with the whole concept of how to love, and how to be loved. I know that if I am whole and fulfilled—which can only be done through Jesus—I should not have all the expectations of my husband that I do. I don't expect him to know that there is a certain way to load a dishwasher that is more effective. I don't expect that he is going to somehow psychically know that something is bothering me. And yet, there is still within me a buried expectation that he will know how to comfort me when I am upset and crying instead of making a chart of all the reasons why I shouldn't be upset. I have to let that go.

My therapist says that I need to communicate what I need from him so that he will have the opportunity to give it, because he does not know what I need. This makes perfect sense to me, but in the midst of intense emotion it is really difficult for me to just say, "Can I please have a hug?" There is a little, snarky voice that wants to add in, "Are you kidding me? Can't you see that I'm hurting and need comfort? Why are you trying to convince me not to be upset?" Quite obviously reaching that stage of acceptance is still a work in progress for me.

After so many years of being in therapy, I am pretty good at discussing issues when I am upset with my partner, and over time, I have learned how to approach situations effectively. However, I'm not so good when my partner is upset with *me*, and bombards me out of the blue. I am still shellshocked from my experience with my previous partner, Pat. He was insane, so no type of communication really worked with him.

The ideal way to deal with conflict is to focus on *feelings* instead of *facts*. You can argue about facts all day, and still never come to a resolution; our egos want to be right and to justify our actions. But feelings are different.

The best way of communicating issues is to lead with something along the lines of, "Honey can I talk to you for a minute?" When you have your partner's attention, then you should sit down and look at each other without distractions. Then you can express your needs with words such as, "I just want to share how I'm feeling. I'm not expecting anything from you, and I love you. When XYZ happened, it left me feeling hurt and angry. I am feeling quite triggered right now, and I am working on dealing with it. I am not blaming you for anything, and you don't need to change anything, but I wanted to let you know how I am feeling.

The ideal response would be, "I hear that you are feeling hurt and angry." Then you should take your partner's hand in yours and look into his or her eyes with all the sincerity you can muster, and say, "I am so sorry you are feeling this way and that my actions contributed to that. I love you and I do not want to ever hurt you." And then leave it.

Later, when the emotions are not as high, if one of you feels the need to explain what happened that led to XYZ, you should talk about it. It may sound easy to implement ... but it is anything *but*.

Sadly, Alberto's way of addressing conflict, delivered in an angry tone, usually while I am in the middle of doing something like cooking dinner, goes something like this. "You did XYZ. It's not right! And this is how a *Christian* behaves? I wouldn't do that to you. You obviously don't care about me. You need someone different than me. You also did ABC, and a few months ago you did EFG and you always do HIJ. You never ...".

Unfortunately, he is fond of 'blaming' words and when this happens, I get angry and defensive, and I try to justify why XYZ didn't really happen that way, and how I don't always do ABC, and I don't even remember EFG. Then he argues, saying I *did* do it ... and back and forth it goes until eventually—perhaps because of my slower-processing, easily overwhelmed brain—I shut down and pull away emotionally. He wants to continue arguing, but I walk away, usually trying to convince myself that I'm not hurt by his accusations.

After a year-and-a-half of marriage, we still do this dance, which is feeding resentment. Lack of effective communication is the cause of break-down in most relationships, and unfortunately we don't know how to communicate properly. A short while ago I found myself consumed with thoughts of, "If only Alberto would do XYZ, then we wouldn't have these problems in our relationship and things would be so much better." Immediately, I noticed I was slipping into my old codependent habits and allowing his moods to affect me way too much. Luckily, I am now able to recognize that it's not really *about* me. His anger and his communication issues belong to him, and are for him to deal with. If he starts to raise his voice to me, I simply say that if he doesn't speak to me respectfully, I will have to distance myself. I am only responsible for the way I communicate, and how I react. This, to me, exemplifies healthy boundaries.

While I've read about interpersonal communication strategies, and learned many of them in counseling, it takes time for them to really sink in and become tools. Cognitively, I understand what needs to happen, and I really *do* want to live this way—not holding onto resentment, communicating effectively with my partner, showing compassion, etc., etc. … but it is so freaking hard! I can do it well enough with the small things, but then there are those game-changing scenarios that come up in relationships that seem impossible to navigate in a way that demonstrates the best version me.

One thing that truly troubles me is that Alberto stopped coming to church and stopped praying with me almost immediately after we got married. I feel betrayed because it was literally THE line in the sand when we began dating. How do I let that go and not have expectations? I expected him to hold true to what he promised when we met. Had I known he was not going to share my faith, there is no way I would have ever dated him—not even if he was the kindest, most handsome, amazing man on the planet. I've tried my best to express my feelings about this to him, but it has changed nothing. There is always some excuse for why he can't go. Another thing that bothers me is that he presented himself as an athletic man and a healthy eater, and he most certainly is *not*. So, I feel he misrepresented himself. While he has a ton of amazing qualities—but those issues would have been deal-breakers for me.

Part of me wants to blame him for misleading me, but I know that I am partially at fault. The truth of the matter is I just took his word at face value and rushed into marriage because I mistakenly thought that by saying he was a Christian, he meant he had the same fire inside him and beliefs as me. I was naive and now I am paying the price. Once again, I made a fantasy version of a man based on what he *told* me without actually allowing myself enough time to really see who he was. I guess the saying holds true that 'old habits die hard'.

There are times that I feel stuck in a marriage to an absolutely wonderful man ... and doubt creeps in that he is not right for me. But I made a vow to God when I married him. No one forced me to get married. I felt certain God had led him to me. I thought all the signs were there. Maybe He did, and part of my story is yet to unfold. I hope so. I could easily blame my decision on my brain injury, saying it has made me impulsive, and so I idealize things. But my naivety doesn't stem from that. My history with men and relationships clearly indicates that I am prone to creating the 'perfect' man in my mind, rather than seeing what stands before me. There is something in me that always wants to see the best in people, and to not acknowledge the bad things. I like to believe that everyone is good until they prove me wrong. Some may call it gullible, but really it's because deep down there is still a girl who wants a fairytale ending.

In therapy, I have been talking about this quite a bit. In my prayers, I have as well. I continually ask God to take negativity and resentment away from my heart and teach me how to forgive Alberto. I remember all those times I was in church, before I married Alberto, learning about God and feeling fulfillment in the love of Jesus. I want to get back to that feeling. I did not need to have a man beside me in order to feel that immense joy, and I don't need it now. But I really expected I would share this wonderful feeling with my life partner—and yet Sunday after Sunday I go to church alone, and my resentment at his lack of interest in sharing this with me grows. I don't want it to be this way for the rest of my life.

My therapist says God can work to make something wonderful out of this. I believe with every fiber of my being that this is true on a spiritual level. However, the human side of me keeps wanting to wallow in misery and imagining a very lonely retirement. Sometimes I think it is lonelier to be with someone, and not able to communicate with that person, than it is to be alone.

As I get older, and retirement looms, I wonder whether I'll have a lonely retirement, which makes me miserable … and the more miserable I get, the more bitterness I feel, and the farther apart Alberto and I grow. Yet when I immerse myself in reading the Bible, pray, go to Bible study, and talk with fellow believers, I know there is hope and that God is working in me—and in Alberto—and that everything is going to be okay. In those moments, I can really love Alberto.

We really are what we feed our thoughts. It sounds cliché, but it really is a day-to-day choice, moment to moment choice. I cannot expect my husband to be someone he is not. I cannot let his moods or words uncenter me. He is a wonderful man who is flawed, like we all are, but I can't expect him to change, nor can I blame him for our issues. My role is to take responsibility for myself and ensure my relationship with God is the utmost priority. Only then can I really be the wife, mother, daughter, and friend that I was made to be.

After all the healing I have done, after all the years of therapy, after all the books I've read, I thought I had things figured out. But I don't. Not even close. I'm learning to see my husband the way God sees him. I'm learning to take that 'step back' in the middle of a disagreement in order to see what is really happening, asking myself … How am I being triggered? How do I really feel? How does my husband feel? How is he being triggered?

We all have a certain degree of fear in us. We don't want to feel hurt. We don't want to feel abandoned. We don't want to really take a deep look in the mirror and recognize our part in things because it is easier to point the finger. We expect our partners to act in a certain way and when they do not, we become disappointed. Michael Jackson quoted it best when he sang, "If you want to make the world a better place, take a look at yourself and make that change," in his hit song, *Man in the Mirror*. It's so easy to say, but so hard to do.

I refuse to run away from myself and distract myself anymore, even though sometimes there is part of me that wants to do this. I don't feel ashamed of who I am, or what I have done in the past. It brought me to today.

Me

My name is Susan, but people call me Suzie. I'm a 45-year-old woman. I'm on my third marriage, though some might call it my fourth if you count the relationship I had with my bipolar, common-law husband, Pat. I have two kids and three step-kids.

I have a progressive incurable life-altering disease called Ankylosing Spondylitis. I struggle every day with chronic pain and fatigue. Ankylosing Spondylitis is an autoimmune disease that makes my body attack all of my joints, and my spine, causing them to fuse and become inflamed. Organs can also be affected. To make matters worse, my spine is crooked and inflamed as well, and I also have some herniated discs. However, while I live with these conditions, they do not own me, or define me.

I take biologics that weaken my immune system to slow the progression of the disease, which means that when I get a common cold, it hits me ten times harder and ten times longer than it does the average person. I go for nerve blocks every week consisting of 30 needs being poked into my face, head and neck. Sometimes I use a cane to ambulate, because the pain from my back radiates down my leg and causes my foot to get numb. Some days my hands are swollen, and I cannot open a jar. Sometimes I can barely move my neck or pick up something from the floor. But I refuse to give in. I walk every day. I go to the gym regularly. There are days when it seems impossible, and I don't want to do anything physical, but I push hard and do it anyway. I always feel better afterward.

Having this disease is like having a bad case of the flu, where your body feels like it has been hit like a truck, combined with constant pain and stiffness. I feel this way all day, every day. It is relentless. I have done my best to get used to the pain, and over time I've developed tolerance that allows me to do the things that need to be done. However, there are days when I just can't cook dinner, so we order in and I don't let myself feel guilty.

When a flare-up hits, it adds a new level of intensity to my pain that sometimes makes me irritable and moody. I try to avoid taking narcotics or opioids to alleviate it, but sometimes I must. I have been on nonsteroidal anti-inflammatory Drugs (NSAIDs) for over 15 years and my stomach has paid the price, so I take them sparingly now. I tried cannabis oil, but turns out I'm allergic to it.

Many people do not understand how hard it is to live with chronic pain, and what it does to every aspect of you, but life goes on and there are days when it is not so bad. I try not to let my suffering affect my mood, but body, mind, and soul are all connected, so it is inevitable. Most people, when they have the flu, feel and act miserable, but I've been sick for so many years that I'm good at pushing my misery aside. If I appear happy, it means I am happy—but often I am also tired or in a lot of pain. This makes it difficult for people to understand how sick I really am. Some days I can go for long walks, while other days I can barely move.

Asking for help is really difficult for me, and it feels like admitting defeat, and so I try hard to distract myself from thinking about the pain and just carry on. Someone asked me once how I deal with so much pain on a constant basis. The answer is that I do it on a moment by moment basis; I seize the moments when the pain is not so bad and make the most of them.

Along with my physical issues, I also have mild lingering effects from a traumatic brain injury that occasionally causes some brain fog and fatigue, especially when I am overwhelmed (which happens easily) or when I'm trying to do too many things at once. I don't do well in crowds and, even though I try, I can no longer multitask. My memory is sketchy, and I have burned more than a couple of pots on the stove because I got distracted and forgot I was cooking.

I have had 22 surgeries, and now can freely admit that I am not Wonder Woman, (even though the urge to take on more than I can handle still creeps in). I am a recovering people pleaser. I am an empath. I feel things very deeply and can be quite sensitive. I will give beyond my limits, and I struggle with boundaries at times. I need alone time to recharge my batteries, and I am grumpy in the mornings because it usually takes a good 30 minutes for the pain to settle down and my joints to start working. Don't talk to me before I've had my coffee!

With all the physical things that have happened in my life I could have easily given up, as my brother Nick did. But God had different plans for me. By showing me the path to Him, I learned to appreciate the small things in life, such as a simple hike in nature, or a paddle board on a lake. These things do so much to uplift my spirits. I still get defensive when I feel I'm being attacked, and I have a tendency to shut down emotionally when I'm hurt and push people away, but I'm working on it. It is a constant daily choice.

I work full time and take care of my dad who lives in another city 35 minutes away. He is 89 and not doing well. I do his shopping and banking, and I arrange all his appointments. He calls me three to four times a day, and every few months there is that dreaded call in the middle of the night because he has fallen, and I have to rush to the hospital to be with him. It's overwhelming at times.

My husband and I fight but I love him and am committed to our marriage. I am glad I married him, because it is teaching me a lot about the person God created me to be versus the person I thought I wanted to be. I have learned that the things my husband says or does should not influence how I conduct myself, or what *I* choose to say and do. I have a responsibility to be true to myself, to establish healthy boundaries, and to act with love and compassion. I am a work in progress, and I have a feeling this learning will be lifelong.

My psychologist painted an analogy for me the other day. She said that we are all like houses with fences around our yards. Each yard has weeds, and some yards have more than others. However, we are only responsible for our own weeds. We cannot expect someone to come to pick ours, nor can we go around trying to help other people with *their* weeds. We can encourage and support each other in the weeding, but we each have to do our own work in our *own* yards.

This resonated deeply with me. I spent my whole life ignoring my weeds, and instead I tried to weed other people's yards, hoping that somehow that would take care of *my* weeds. I looked for a man to make my weeds go away. That strategy does not work!.

My mother and I have a good relationship now. She has found someone to share her life with. She's happy, and has been working on her 'yard'. She still worries about me, and I wish she wouldn't, but that is her choice. Last year she had a knee replacement, and I got to witness what a strong fighter she is. My respect for her grew immensely. She followed the doctor's recommendations word for word and diligently did her exercises so she would heal as fast as possible. She was back at work within three months, taking a one-hour bus trip downtown at four in the morning, at the age of 73, to work as a marketing consultant. She just retired after sustaining a concussion from a fall and is healing well.

My father is slowly dying. He spent his life running away from his 'yard' and now he is housebound, staring at the weeds. He is depressed. I do what I can to help with his physical needs, and keep him company, but sadly he does not carry the fighting spirit, and I'm not sure whether he ever did. Unfortunately, he *does* carry around a lot of guilt, and he sees himself as a poor, helpless, old man. There is no physical reason why he cannot do more than he does, but mentally he is manifesting a lifetime of repressed feelings. It is heartbreaking to watch.

There are four teenagers in my house, along with a toddler, a cat, and a dog. The teenagers are trying; my eldest daughter has attention-deficit/hyperactivity disorder (ADHD), and doesn't like me right now. If I tell her that the sun is shining, she will argue with me that it is black. We argue a lot because she lies to me and sneaks out of the house, and I recently found a bag of marijuana and birth control pills in her drawer while I was cleaning her room. I can't be too hard on her though; she is the product of a mother who had no self-esteem for much of her life. I pray one day she will be ready to go to counseling and talk to me.

Just like my parents, I did the best I could with both my children and myself, and every day I try to learn to do better. I carry some guilt about the tumultuous life they have had, and I wish I knew when my kids were babies what I know now. But feeling guilty doesn't solve anything. At the very least, my children know how loved they are.

My youngest stepson, who has a very strong personality, also has ADHD. He cries when he doesn't get what he wants, often many times a day, and he likes to hit and play rough. I know now why God gave me girls because I really struggle with this kid. He is cute and smart, but he is exhausting. Maybe it's because I'm older and don't have the energy I used to, or maybe it's that I'm not used to having a little boy around. Either way, I am committed to being the best mother and stepmother I know how to be.

There are times when the pain, fatigue and feeling of being overwhelmed are too much to bear and I need to cry, and so I allow myself 'two - three tears' and then pull myself together. There are moments when I feel hopeless, and I want to bury myself under my covers. I allow myself ten minutes and move on. In my mind, there is no alternative.

When I was young, I was the girl who was always on the go. I got my scuba diving license at 17, and I rock climbed, skydived, paraglided, white-water rafted, and jogged regularly. I was always active and on the go. It is overwhelming to think of all of the things I can't do anymore, and contemplate the broken body I have been left with. I could really sink into a deep depression if I allowed myself to, but I chose to focus on the things that I CAN do, and be truly grateful for them. God can, and is, doing wonderful things in me. He did not create all of my suffering, but he has used my life experiences and experiences I have labelled as 'bad' or 'negative, for good. Even when I can't see His purpose in the moment, I wholly and completely trust it.

I am grateful every day that I can walk, and I choose not to focus on the fact that I cannot run or dance like I used to. Yes, I have the occasional pity party, complete with champagne and balloons, but I strive to focus on the beautiful things I have been given, from my home and family to the fact that I can still spell my name—and everything in between. In life, there are always those who have it better, and those who have it worse. I think I am somewhere in the middle. This is the life that was gifted to me, and I am grateful for every single thing that has happened in my life, not just the good things, because it is the compilation of experiences that brought me here.

In my job as an insurance professional, I listen to clients cry about how much their life has changed because of their car accident and subsequent brain injury, pain, or other issue, and I truly empathize with them. It makes me grateful for God's guidance, and reinforces that everything in my life happened the way it did so I could grow. I am who I am now as a result of it. I found faith, hope, and freedom.

People affected by traumatic events, such as a loved one's suicide, a life-altering disease or a big surgery, with God's grace gravitate toward me. When they find me, I can walk with them and hold their hand. I can listen with understanding and compassion because I've been there myself. A few weeks ago, a woman who had to have a hip replacement at a young age approached me and told me her situation made her feel very alone. Sharing my experience with her brought her a great amount of comfort, and also provided her with some important information. When my father went for his first heart surgery, I was able to console him and ease his fear.

The point is this; I got through everything that happened and through it all I came to understand that my suffering was not just about my own growth, but was preparation to help others. There are no words to describe how blessed I feel. No one could have fixed my problems for me, just as I cannot solve other people's problems as I once believed I could. Sometimes all we need is to feel understood, and that someone cares.

My children may not listen to me much of the time, but they witness and see everything I do. They learn by watching, not by what they are told. When they are old enough, they will know what perseverance, love, and forgiveness look like. They will know what it looks like to be grateful for what you have and *can* do, not resentful for not what you *don't* have or *can't* do.

There is so much more that God has in store for me. He is working in my heart right now. He trained me and is preparing me for all that is yet to come. I know that Alberto is my perfect partner here in this life because I have placed my faith and trust in God. I reflect on the time when Alberto and I met and, at the time, I really was convicted that our meeting was divinely orchestrated. I choose to believe that, and I know the Lord will continue working in both of us to give us a healthy marriage.

Mostly, the biggest thing about my life journey is that I found love I never thought was possible in God. There is no longer an empty seat beside me; instead, it is filled with an all-encompassing love composed of grace and forgiveness. It is a love that never lets me down even in the hardest of times. It is a love that has always been there, and always will be. It is the love of God. None of the other stuff really matters. It is the answer to all of my questions that I had. I am a child of God. He loves me so much that He died for me. Nothing in this life can take away the fact that I will be with Him when I die, and He alone is my happily ever after.

One Day at a Time

I wake up to the sound of a door closing. My husband has left for work, I'm guessing. I reach over and grab my phone to look at the time. There are still 25 minutes before I have to get up. I want to sleep more because I feel so exhausted, but the pain in my back won't let me get comfortable, so I toss and turn. I feel irritated. I would love to wake up feeling rested and not have any pain. My joints feel stiff and achy, but getting out of bed seems like too much effort so I linger.

The alarm wakes me up and I stagger out of bed to the kitchen and push the button to make coffee, something my wonderful husband has already set up. I have to remember to thank him for that. A hot cup of an acidic substance in the morning isn't exactly best for the body, but I love it and I need it to wake up. The pain starts to dull with my clumsy slow movements, and so I slump into my office chair and boot up my computer. It's 6:30 a.m. Outside, my office window reveals a cloudy grey sky that is reflective of my mood. It's technically still summer, but it has been an unseasonably cool one. I feel ripped off, because I spend nine months of the year waiting for the hot summer sun to warm my ever-cold body. And now it's over.

School has just started back, and soon my youngest daughter, Samantha, will be awake soon. Mary, my eldest, just moved out last week to go to university. I can't even think about that without crying so I try to push the thought away, but tears well up anyway and spill over my unwashed face. People say to cherish the younger years of your children because they go by so quickly, and it is true. It seems like just a short while ago she was a little girl who followed me around everywhere. Now she is living on campus, and couldn't be happier to be on her own. All I can think of is the word 'bittersweet'. At least there won't be any arguing in the mornings as I make sure she is out of bed and not late again, like she was 32 times last semester. Mary was never one to follow rules.

I miss the girl who needed me and actually wanted to hang around me. People say that eventually teenagers come back once they have experienced the real world. Here's hoping. The last couple of years, she barely grumbled a hello to me except for when she needed something, like money or the car. When my children were younger, on a gloomy day like today we would bury ourselves under the covers, making them into a fort, and sing songs. I know it's time for her to spread her wings and lead her own life, but it is hard not to feel sad. I suppose most parents go through this when their child leaves home. Mary's strong will and independence will see her through and, in the end, I'm happy as long as she's happy.

The last year with Mary was particularly challenging. I found out she was sneaking out of the house after we were all sound asleep, probably to go out with her new boyfriend and get high, and I when I was folding her clothes one day, I found a bag of weed and birth control pill tucked away in the back of her drawer. There is a small part of me, to this day, that wants me to feel like a failure as a parent, but I know to nip that thought in the bud and not allow it to go any further. I did the best I could with what I knew at the time, and I never intentionally set out to do them any wrong, just as my parents never meant to harm my brother and I. It is easy to have thoughts of, "If only I knew then what I know now, things would be different," but that does not solve anything.

It's time to focus. As I do every morning at work, I complete some meaningless tasks that don't require much brain function until the caffeine kicks in. When I hear Samantha's alarm clock at 7:00 a.m., I go and make sure she's awake. She is up already, and seeing her fills my heart with love. Like her sister, she is the tallest girl in her class, and I think she had another growth spurt this past summer. Unlike her sister, she doesn't argue with me at all. She is kind and so sweet, although as the lure of social media is increases, she spends a lot of time on her phone.

My thoughts drift to all the years that have slipped away. I wish I had been a better role model. I wish I had been the type of mother they both deserve. The path of self-recrimination, and wallowing in self-pity, is like a fork in the road in front of me. *Nope, I'm not taking that road right now. Focus Suzie!*

After dropping Samantha off at the bus stop, it's time to go back to work. A few hours go by, and it has been a good and productive morning—but I got so absorbed in my work that I forgot to get up and walk around to ease my back pain. The fact that I got so distracted and lost track of time is irritating because now there is a price to be paid.

I'm a claims adjuster for an insurance company. Claims adjusters usually get a bad rap, and some think it's a thankless job, but it involves working with severely injured people, which allows my medical knowledge to be put to use. Also, the pay is decent, and I get to work from home, which is what keeps me there. This morning, I'm engrossed in the job because there are a couple of interesting cases that were just given to me, and this is the part of the job that I love. I am very good at taking messy situations and turning them around, and although there are many aspects of my job that I could do without, I really love knowing that I am helping people.

The pain in my back is increasing now, and I have no idea how I'm going to sit at my desk for one minute longer. I told myself yesterday that I would not take another Tramadol, which is an opiod based pain reliever used to treat moderate to severe pain in adults, but I really want to. Alberto mentioned yesterday that I seem more irritable than usual, and that he thinks it's the pills. This may be true. Since my fall in the backyard three weeks ago, a new level of pain has engulfed me, and that's why I've taken these drugs.

So, I'm left with a choice: Do I endure the pain? Or do I take the pill so I can continue to sit, but risk being irritable?

Down goes a pill, followed by a glass of lukewarm water. My disease causes me to feel cold much of the time, so cold water is out of the question.

In walks frustration hand in hand with irritability. The meds will take up to an hour to take effect, but until they do it's annoying that I can't do the things I want to do. I hate this disease. I hate that it makes me want to crawl out of my skin sometimes. I hate how it affects my mood. I can't want to be in Heaven. I don't want my life to end, I just can't wait for the suffering to stop. It's so unfair. Haven't I suffered enough?

The worst part is that there is no cure. I am only likely to get worse—and then what? What will my life look like then? My eyes start to well up with tears. It's so tiring to put on a happy face while my back feels like there are hot pokers in my spine. The escape and joy I found in painting and playing the piano have been stripped away just like dancing and jogging were. The depression feels like a tidal wave about to crash over me. Any awareness I usually have that entertaining these thoughts will create a depressive snowball effect is gone. All I can think is, *this stinks!*

Sitting for prolonged periods is poison, and I know I should probably walk around, but I don't want to. I want to wallow in self-pity and groan at the injustice of my disease and how it has ravaged my body. The reflection in the mirror shows how much I have aged these last few years. The constant pain, and barrage of medications and surgeries—not to mention my history of relationship drama—has taken its toll.

Slumping on the couch, I stare at the wall contemplating what to do. I can feel the drug slowly start to work and my anger slowly subsides. *Pull yourself together Suzie*, I tell myself. *You can do this.* This disease is not going to ruin my life, I decide. Distractions sometimes work, so I pick up a vacuum and start cleaning. I may be sick, but at least the house will be clean.

Soon, I can get back to work; however fatigue has now taken up residence in my body, and it feels like a ton of bricks strapped onto each bone. People think fatigue means being tired, but disease-related fatigue means feeling like you have the flu, and being so weak and exhausted that you can't see straight. The bed beckons me relentlessly, but I won't give in. *God, please give me the strength to get through this day.* Oh yes, God! I forgot to pray today. It bewilders me that the very thing that brings me peace and joy, I keep forgetting to do! So I say a quick prayer.

After praying, my spirits feel a little lighter. I feel that going for a walk will help me, but it feels like an impossible task. Coffee will make my stomach feel worse, but the alternative of calling in sick to work again and sinking into the couch in front of the TV will only make me feel useless. The dog looks up at me and pokes my leg; she wants to go out, so there is my answer. Putting on running shoes is more effort than I can handle, so I go with the ever-fashionable socks and sandals. I am Canadian after all.

As I head outside, there is a cool, light breeze and the sun is trying to break through the clouds. Our cat appears out of nowhere and follows us down the driveway onto the street. The cat likes to go on walks with us, and lets out howls when we go too fast. This always makes me chuckle, and I begin to feel a little less encumbered. I love our neighborhood. The large lots and houses that were built in the 1950s have a unique country charm to them—our neighbourhood is not quite rural, but pretty close. When there is a westerly wind, we get a whiff of farm life … which I have still not quite gotten used to.

A particularly large tree catches my attention, and once again I am filled with awe at the beauty of it. *Thank you, God, for creating such beauty!* Often we are so caught up and busy that we don't even notice how much life and wonder is in a single tree. It touches me to my core, putting my pain and fatigue in the background. Through the stormy winter winds, this tree survived naked and exposed, and now it is lush and majestic. Birds and squirrels have made their nests in it. In a month or two the leaves will fall off and it will be bare again ... and then the cycle will repeat.

I think life is kind of like that. Sometimes it is full and beautiful with so many possibilities, and then the cold comes and before you know it, you are naked, exposed and seemingly dead ... only to once again slowly re-build, a little bigger than before. This may sound like a simplistic viewpoint; obviously, life is much more complicated, but nevertheless there is some truth in there. Obviously, philosophy is not my strong suit.

By now the tramadol is doing its thing, and returning to work is not that hard. I become immersed in my work again until the phone rings. It's my dad and he is feeling depressed. His voice is barely a whisper as he tells me that he has run out of butter. Then he says he is just waiting for his life to end, and he feels useless because he is not getting any better. He reminds me that his wife left him, and his only living child moved far away, so he has no one.

I know it's just frustration and depression talking, so I don't take this unintentional jab personally. The old Suzie would have gotten defensive and upset at his comment, but if I were in his shoes, I would feel frustrated and alone too. It is not easy to live alone and yet not be totally independent.

I remind him that he is still living at home, where he wants to be, and that he can still walk. There are senior citizens who cannot even do that. I tell him God has a purpose for his life, even in the minimalized state it is in now that he's older, and that although his situation is not what he would like it to be, he should focus on being grateful for what he has. He agrees with me, and his spirits seem somewhat lifted. Experience has taught me that this is the kind of talk he needs. While it hurts me to see that he has no fight left in him, the reality is that he is 89 years old and his heart is failing. I don't know if I would feel any different in his shoes. I wish he'd remarried so he would at least have a companion.

The plan had always been that when my parents got older and needed help, they would come and live with me. After training in palliative care, and volunteering in nursing homes, I told myself that I would *never* put my parents in a home. But after one of my dad's heart surgeries last year, he stayed with us for six weeks and I wound up changing my mind. It was extremely difficult for me to come to that conclusion, but he needs so much attention and care that I just can't do it.

When he stayed with us for those six weeks, I was trying to work during the day, which proved to be very challenging. During that time, I barely spoke with my kids, except to ask them to do chores, and my husband and I were like two ships passing in the night. I realized that they need me too.

It was a tough pill to swallow when I came to the realization that I simply could not look after my dad. In fact, I cannot even look after myself sometimes. I registered him for long term care, and he continues to live in his apartment (which he prefers anyway) while we wait for a placement, which could take years, and meanwhile I keep praying that that I have the strength to do what needs to be done.

This approach is a big step for me, as old Suzie would have tried to do everything for everyone, and then felt guilty when I could not. This new 'boundaries' thing is awesome! I do what I can to help, but I make sure I take care of myself in the process. It is a simple concept that only took 40 years to comprehend and put into practice.

After I finish work, I open up my Bible and read a few verses, but nothing is really seeping in today. I pick up Samantha from the bus stop and she tells me of her day at school. It is such a blessing that she feels comfortable talking to me about everything. I cherish our relationship, although it makes me sad that Mary and I were never that close. I suggest to her that we could play some basketball or something and she agrees.

Once we get inside, I sit on the couch and wait for her to get ready, but suddenly another tidal wave of fatigue comes flooding in, this one much heavier than before. I guess we won't be playing basketball after all. Samantha walks into the room, takes one look at me and tells me we should watch a show instead. I want to cry from the sheer beauty of her heart, and her compassion and perceptiveness. I'm too tired to feel bad about letting her down—but then again, she loves watching movies.

When my batteries are somewhat recharged, it's time to think about dinner. I'm a disaster in the kitchen, and it doesn't help matters that cooking is something I am not fond of. I get to work and then my dad calls again. He sounds a little better, and tells me again that he has run out of butter. The other line beeps in and the support worker tells me she is going to be late, so I call my dad back to let him know. Then he tells me he has run out of diabetic test strips for his little machine, so I have to call the pharmacy to get them to deliver more.

As I'm searching the fridge, hoping for a dinner option to suddenly materialize, Alberto arrives home from work, exhausted from another stressful day. I worry about him because his stress at work consumes him completely, and he struggles to let it go. Even on weekends, he is thinking about work. It's difficult for me to comprehend this, because as soon as I leave my office I don't give work another thought until I am paid to do so again.

Alberto heads to the couch for a nap and Samantha walks into the kitchen to tell me she needs some supplies for school. We still have enough time to go shopping before dinner, and I decide to defrost some spaghetti sauce I cooked a few weeks before and saved.

We head out, and when we pull into the plaza parking lot, I forget why we are there and ask Samantha. She tells me she needs retractable pencils. I try to turn off the car, but it won't turn off. I have left the car in drive, so of course it won't turn off (this happens all too often).

Laughing it off, we get what we need and quickly head home. Alberto is heating the sauce and boiling the noodles, and I'm grateful. We chat for a bit in the kitchen, but I have trouble focusing on what he is saying. His lips are moving and there is sound coming out of his mouth, but my brain isn't processing the information. My neck hurts and the back pain has come back, but I'm unable to express this because I am so darn exhausted. I grumble something and he looks offended, but at this moment I don't care. Everything seems hazy, and curling up on the kitchen floor seems enticing. Somehow, I set the table and we eat.

Slowly, the fog in my head dissipates enough that participation in the conversation is possible. Samantha helps clean up the kitchen, and then heads upstairs to chat with her friends. Alberto seems a little distant and I sense an angry energy. I wonder, *should try to figure out if it was something I said or did?* I decide that if he is upset, he will tell me and then I will apologize for being spaced out when he was speaking with me.

Still, I'm not quite satisfied with leaving it to chance, so I ask how he is doing. He says he is okay, and so I let it go. Old Suzie would have pressed him to tell me what was bothering him, because it would have upset me not to know. I may even have gotten irritated at the thought that he was upset with me. This incident, though benign, gets me thinking. I know that I still try to put on a face of being 'okay' even when I am not okay. But I get so tired of hearing myself say that my back hurts, or that I am tired. It's almost as if I don't want to admit to *myself* how I really feel, so I distract myself and pretend that I'm okay. I don't want to be 'that woman with a disability'. Then again, by being this way I'm ignoring all the work I have done on acceptance and being honest.

In those moments when fatigue and pain overtake me, it is so hard to snap out of it, but for me it's even harder to say simple words such as, "Hey honey, I'm not feeling the greatest right now, but I really want to hear what you have to say so can we talk a little later?" Maybe I should start meditating again.

I seek out Alberto who is watching TV and say that I'm sorry if I wasn't paying attention to what he was saying earlier, because I wasn't feeling the greatest. "No problem," he says. He needs time to process, so I leave him be.

Samantha and I watch a movie, and then it's time for bed. We hold hands and say prayers like we have done every night since she was born. The day feels like a blur. Heck, my life feels like a blur most of the time.

It's all very routine, and it makes me wonder, *so what exactly is the point of life?* I ponder this as I lay down to sleep. Millions of people have asked the same question and, depending on your beliefs, there are a million different answers. I am 'perfectly imperfectly made', and there is a purpose to it all that I will never fully comprehend. What if I was made just to love? So many years I've spent waiting to feel loved, and now that I do sharing it and giving it can only bring joy. I lean over and kiss my husband goodnight. I'll do better tomorrow.

Today I have to drive into the city for a case conference for a client. I decided to sneak in a chiropractic appointment on the way. The only decent chiropractor I've found is in the city. I have tried numerous others, but they just do not compare. I am looking forward to a bit of pain relief.

The highway is moving at a steady pace and normally I listen to the radio, but I am struck by an overwhelming feeling to pray for my family. Typically I pray for them at night time but the urge is so strong to pray for their protection right now that I do. I am not sure if it is my husband or my daughters that I am praying for, but I have a feeling like something bad is going to happen. *Please God, if anything bad is meant to happen, let it only be minor and not severe.* I pray this over and over again until I feel enough peace that I can stop.

Roughly 30 minutes later, I am finished with the chiropractor and am feeling a bit of relief. I get into my car to head to my work appointment. My phone rings. It's Alberto. He tells me he has had an accident at work, but he is okay. I can hear in his voice that he is concerned, but trying not to worry me. He said a piece of equipment fell on his head and he fell to the ground. He was not knocked unconscious, but he has a headache. His boss told him to go to the doctor, and he told me he was on his way. He doesn't sound like himself. I tell him to go home and that I will meet him there. I cancel my meeting and do my best to rush home.

When I see my husband, though there is no gaping wound or blood rushing, I can tell that Alberto is a bit dazed and confused. He shows me the picture of the piece of equipment that had fallen on his head. It is a 15-pound, long, rectangular piece of metal. I know right away that my prayers were answered, because as bad as it was, he got hit by the blunt, flat side instead of a corner or an edge. If he'd been hit by one of the sharp corners, things would have ended a lot differently.

As I drive Alberto to the hospital, I quietly thank God that this was not more serious. We wait for six hours, and thankfully there is no brain damage, but he definitely has a concussion and maybe some nerve damage. As we sit and wait for discharge papers, I can't help but see the irony of the situation. Brian suffered a concussion just one month before I met him. Pat had a significant head injury a few months after we started dating. I've experienced many concussions, and a brain injury. Two of my closest friends have head injuries. My mom just had a mild concussion not that long ago. And finally, I have spent the last 20 years working with brain-injured clients and taking courses and certifications on head injuries. And now here I sat with my husband, envisioning the road ahead as he heals.

Sweet merciful Lord, what are you trying to teach me? Is this what you have prepared me for? Could this be the thing that brings Alberto and I closer together, or closer to You, dear Lord?

The answer will come if I do the absolute best thing: Pray, love, trust and have faith.

We all come to a point in our story when we stop to take a pause and look at the journey behind us and try to make sense of it. The trials we face, though they can be torturous, are also what make life worth living.

Life can be complicated and exhausting, but it is also rich and invigorating!

www.ingramcontent.com/pod-product-compliance
Lightning Source LLC
LaVergne TN
LVHW041636060526
838200LV00040B/1592